# Functional Aids
# for the
# Multiply
# Handicapped

Edited by

# Isabel P. Robinault, Ph.D.

Supervisor, Research Utilization Laboratory
ICD Rehabilitation and Research Center
New York, New York

Formerly Coordinator, Professional Activities
United Cerebral Palsy Associations, Inc.
New York, New York

This publication was made possible in
part through the generosity of
the Smith, Kline & French Foundation,
Philadelphia, Pennsylvania.

# Functional Aids for the Multiply Handicapped

Prepared under the auspices of the
United Cerebral Palsy Associations, Inc.

Medical Department
Harper & Row, Publishers
Hagerstown, Maryland
New York, Evanston, San Francisco, London

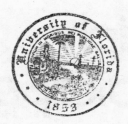

STANDARD BOOK NUMBER: 06-142276-2

LIBRARY OF CONGRESS CATALOG CARD NUMBER:
75-189635

*To the challengers and the challenged*
*whose initiative is recorded in this book*

# Contents

# Preface

This resource book is the outgrowth of many years of inquiry and exchange between personnel of the United Cerebral Palsy Associations and individuals with multiple disabilities, their parents, contact-care personnel, and personnel of clinics, schools, and other helping agencies. Each year we receive hundreds of questions asking what to use, where to buy it, or how to construct an item that would enable its user to function more independently or to live in a more meaningful way. Answering these questions became an unwieldy task because of their number and the paucity of published information. There are excellent resources for individuals with muscular weakness or joint impairments, but these were not found to be generally applicable to the unharnessed strength, the random motions, or the multiple disabilities of the cerebral palsied individual.

We discovered that answers did exist all over the United States, but no one had organized them. Therefore, we asked a Committee of Consultants to review the hundreds of photographs, diagrams, and descriptions submitted by commercial companies, private individuals, clinics, schools, camps, and members of the helping professions. Functional aids and equipment were selected from these to cover the developmental range from infancy to maturity. The final selection was grouped into four parts: transfer, travel, and mobility; personal care; communications and learning; and recreation.

The questions that prompted us to write this book come from three groups and we have included information to aid all three. For individuals with cerebral palsy and their parents, there are many common-sense items which are readily available on the general market. Other information should be particularly suited to the needs of contact-care personnel, of therapy clinics, day-care and developmental centers, special schools, camps, etc. Resources and alternative procedures for enhancing function will hopefully fulfill the special purposes of physicians, therapists, nurses, homemaker personnel, and education, recreation, and rehabilitation specialists, as well as professional educators in the field.

Equipment should be selected for the individual or specific individuals who will use it. In its selection, one should keep in mind the goal which the equipment is to serve. Equipment should not be ordered until the users and the program are established. We have given precautions for almost every item since it is *how* a piece of equipment is used that makes it functional. Each item was originally made for a specific individual, and if it cannot be made to order, it will have to be adapted to the use of another specific individual.

Major service organizations that had published materials related to these areas, or to this population, were contacted, and they contributed many items of special relevance. They, and every other contributor, have been individually credited throughout the book, not only to acknowledge their cooperation but to provide the reader with pertinent resources for any related questions that may arise. At the end of the book we have appended a list of these sources with their addresses. Since we began this book, many of these manufacturers and organizations have moved or changed their name. We have endeavored to keep all names and addresses current and to properly acknowledge all sources, but due to the very large number of contributors, we may have inadvertently made a mistake. If so, we offer our sincere apologies.

If this book is a true response to the hundreds of inquiries of the past years, it will enable individuals with multiple disabilities to avoid being handicapped by their condition and should contribute toward more functional and meaningful lives.

New York

I.P.R.

# Acknowledgments

The United Cerebral Palsy Associations, Inc., wish to acknowledge and thank the volunteer Committee of Consultants who worked with the Editor on this resource book for over three years. They reviewed hundreds of items and tried out many functional aids whose prior analyses had seemed superficial. They are to be credited with the precautions, the guidelines for use, the alternatives of choice in cases of purchase and the review of construction diagrams. As a group, the consultants do not agree on all items included in this book. However, each respects a valid difference of opinion which may result from experience gained with populations of varying functional capacities. Therefore, the Editor has included some selections justified by individual experience.

The members of this committee have contributed a cumulative "know-how" that will help children to reach their potentialities and help adults with multiple disabilities to make the most of their capabilities. Therefore, we thank and salute:

**Robert Bartlett,** R.P.T., Associate Professor and Chairman, Program in Physical Therapy, Downstate Medical Center, Brooklyn, New York

**Patricia H. Buehler,** O.T.R., Consultant, Spastic Children's Foundation; Consultant, United Cerebral Palsy Association; Consultant, Development Centers for Handicapped Minors, Los Angeles, California

**Beatrice Crowder,** O.T.R., Formerly of United Cerebral Palsy of Pennsylvania

**Gerry Fullan,** R.N., Formerly of Spastic Aid of Alabama, Birmingham, Alabama

**Una Haynes,** R.N., Associate Director, Professional Services Program Department, United Cerebral Palsy Associations, Inc., New York, New York

**Jay Schleichkorn,** R.P.T., Associate Professor; Director, Program of Physical Therapy, Health Sciences Center, State University of New York, Stony Brook, New York

**Martha Schnebly,** O.T.R., Ed.D., Chief, Occupational Therapy Department, Institute of Rehabilitation Medicine, New York, New York

**Anita Slominski,** O.T.R., Director, Cerebral Palsy Unit, Indiana University Medical School, Indianapolis, Indiana

**Helen Spencer Svirsky,** R.P.T., Supervising Physical Therapist, Alameda County Health Service Agency, San Francisco, California

Illustrations were drawn by **Janet Green.**

# Functional Aids for the Multiply Handicapped

# I
# TRANSFER, TRAVEL, AND MOBILITY

# 1

# Sitting and Standing Equipment

Sitting and standing are means of changing position that have remedial values for the individual with cerebral palsy: They facilitate care, stimulate body function, and place the individual in correct positions for recreational, educational, and therapeutic activities.

## General Precautions

1. Measure the chair and the child, allowing for growth in height and width.
2. Use sturdy materials that can be cleaned.
3. Be sure the base of each item is wide enough to avoid tipping.
4. Use only lead-free paint on any equipment or toys for children.
5. Do not use curved plywood seats that make sitter's legs adduct.
6. Do not let child's feet dangle; if necessary, use nonskid footrests or footstools.
7. Do not put pressure on the back of the head if it accentuates extensor thrust.
8. If sitting balance is poor and extensor thrust is prominent, make seats or seat inserts at an angle so that the child is bent more at the hips than the usual 90-degree sitting position.

9. If the chair is not pushed against a table, provide a lapboard or tray to give security, to give stability by supporting the arms, and to allow for activities.
10. Be sure that the stand-in table has a wide base that cannot be tipped, regardless of direction in which the child leans.
11. Be sure that the table's surface is large enough for activities within the arm reach of the user.
12. Provide locks that cannot be opened accidentally or on purpose by the occupant. Possible solutions for this are two locks, locks below the child's reach, or hook locks.
13. Provide drilled holes or screening in the box section of the table to allow for circulation of air.
14. Have adjustable foot shelves to allow for varied heights.

As to whether the equipment should be constructed or purchased, suitability and/or availability will be the determining factors. In the following pages, diagrams for construction will be given and manufactured items that have proved useful will be presented.

## MEASUREMENTS FOR SPECIAL EQUIPMENT

All measurements for equipment should be taken when the child is fully clothed. A yardstick, not a cloth tape, should be used. In the following list of dimensions to be measured, the letters in parentheses denote the measurements illustrated in Figures 1-1 through 1-4.

Distance from seat to top of head (*A*). This distance (Fig. 1-1) gives the minimal height of the backrest for a child needing full head support (upright or tilted). In practice, it is best to make the backrest 6 inches longer to allow for growth.

Distance from seat to top of shoulders (*B*). This distance is the minimal height of the backrest if shoulder support only is required. If side supports are needed for the head, the bottom edges of the supports must be above this level to give shoulder clearance. Allowance should be made for growth.

Depth of seat (*C*). The measurement should be made with the child's buttocks against the chair back. The seat should be deep enough to support the thighs but should not cut into the back of the knees. There should be a space the width of two fingers between the back of the knees and the end of the seat. To state this another way: The measurement should go from the buttocks to within 1 or 2 inches of the bend of the knee. Check for scoliosis or a dislocated hip, and use the measurement of the *shorter* thigh.

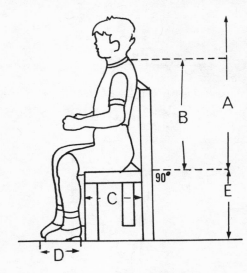

**FIG. 1-1.** Measuring for chair, from seat to top of head, *A;* from seat to top of shoulders, *B;* depth of seat, *C;* depth of footrest, *D;* and distance from seat to footrest, *E.* (Courtesy of United Cerebral Palsy of New York State, adapted from the original prepared by the British Council of Welfare of Spastics)

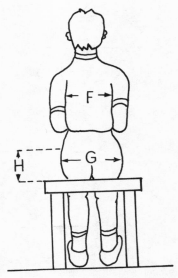

**FIG. 1-2.** Determining width of chair and height of side supports by measuring across the shoulders, *F;* across the hips, *G;* and from seat to elbow, *H.* (Courtesy of United Cerebral Palsy of New York State, adapted from the original prepared by the British Council of Welfare of Spastics)

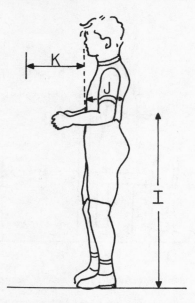

**FIG. 1-3.** Measuring for table, from floor to elbow when standing, *I;* body thickness, *J,* to determine depth of cutout; and forward reach, *K.* (Courtesy of United Cerebral Palsy of New York State, adapted from the original prepared by the British Council of Welfare of Spastics )

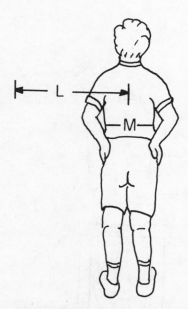

**FIG. 1-4.** Determining width of table by measuring sideways reach from spine, *L;* and width of cutout by body width at elbow, *M.* (Courtesy of United Cerebral Palsy of New York State, adapted from the original prepared by the British Council of Welfare of Spastics )

Depth of footrest (*D*). The footrest should be deep enough to support the whole length of the foot with the shins at right angles to the thighs. The foot must also be at right angles to the shins, *never* in foot-drop position. Some individuals, however, need some dorsiflexion, the degree of which should be determined by optimal function.

Distance from seat to footrest (*E*). The height of the footrest is very important. The foot should be fully supported, but the thighs must not be lifted from the seat.

Width across shoulders (*F*). The backrest should be wide enough to support the whole of the back but should allow for free movement of the arms (Fig. 1-2).

Width across hips (*G*). This measurement should be made while the child is seated. If side support is needed, the child should fit snugly between the side pieces. Since allowance should be made for growth, temporary boards should be fitted inside the fixed ones to reduce the seat width to the required measurement. These boards can be replaced with thinner ones and finally discarded as the child grows.

Distance from seat to elbow (*H*). Side supports should be 1 inch less than this measurement to give clearance for the elbows and to allow the chair to slip under the table. Table or desk surfaces should be 1 inch higher than the elbows to give support to the arms.

If desired, the seat, side supports, and back of the chair may be upholstered with half-inch-thick foam rubber covered with leather cloth. Allowance must be made for this when measurements are taken. In deciding upon upholstering, certain precautions are advisable: A child who perspires freely may be more comfortable without foam and plastic padding. However, side supports for the head should always be upholstered.

Distance from floor to elbow when standing (*I*). This measurement (Fig. 1-3), plus 1 inch, gives the height of the surface of a stand-in table from the floor or platform on which the child stands.

Thickness of body, front to back, at elbow level (*J*). The depth of the cutout from the front edge of the table is determined by this measure.

Length of forward reach measured from chest (*K*). The minimal depth of the table top, measured from the cutout, should equal this measure.

Length of sideways reach measured from spine (*L*). To encourage full use of reach, the width of the table should be twice this measurement (Fig. 1-4).

Width of body at elbow level (*M*). This measurement indicates how wide the cutout should be.

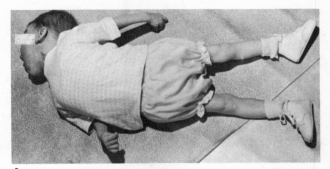

**A**

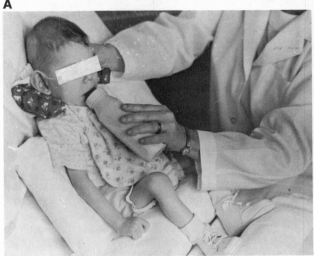

**B**

**FIG. 1-5.** Child with marked extensor thrust (*A*), propped up with sandbags and cut-out neck pillow (*B*) to facilitate feeding. (From Haynes, U. Nursing approaches in cerebral dysfunction. *Amer J Nurs* 68:10:2170–2176 Oct., 1966. Reproduced with permission.)

## SIMPLE SITTING SUPPORTS FOR FUNCTIONAL POSITIONS

For the child with marked extensor thrust Fig. 1-5*A*), a sitting support placed on the bed is helpful. In addition, sandbags will hold the child's feet in dorsiflexion and make secure side supports, if necessary (Fig. 1-5*B*). A neck pillow reduces the pressure on the back of the head. Without it, the pressure encourages the thrusting tendency. Properly fitted shoes on a nonwalker help reduce unwanted stimulus to the feet and sometimes help reduce extensor thrust when the child is in a supported sitting position. In Figure 1-5*B*, the child is not sucking air since a nipple straw draws

liquid from the bottom of the bottle (see section on Sucking Aids for Sitting-Up Feeding in Chapter 5).

## SEATING AIDS FOR SMALL CHILD

### SIMPLE PROPPING DEVICES

For short-term sitting positions for children, use sandbags, firm pillows, rubber tires, boxes, or crates for extra support. A rubber tire often makes a satisfactory seat. Place the child tailor-fashion (Indian style) in the tire (Fig. 1-6), and use firm pillows or sandbags for low-back and side support, if needed. A cut-out board may be placed over the tire as a table to hold the toys.

### Precautions

1. Do not let the child lie in bed for extended periods during the day. He should not face a blank wall or high bolster-padded protector. Mobiles and stimulating toys should be available within the child's visual and tactile fields.
2. Before the child is transferred to an appropriate chair, prop him in a sitting position for a time, with firm pillows and sandbags for support.

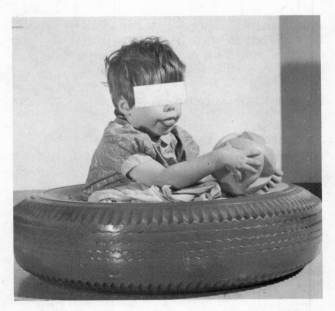

**FIG. 1-6.** Automobile tire used as prop, in which child is comfortably seated tailor fashion. (Courtesy of United Cerebral Palsy of Greater Detroit)

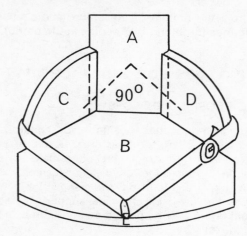

**FIG. 1-7.** Diagram for constructing Knickerbocker corner seat. (Courtesy of Maj. B. Knickerbocker, Army Hospital, Fort Dix, N.J.)

3. Letting the child sit tailor-fashion helps counteract extreme back tension. Do this for just a few minutes at first; then the time may be extended to 15 to 20 minutes at a sitting.

## THE KNICKERBOCKER CORNER SEAT

The Knickerbocker corner seat (Fig. 1-7) is easily constructed for small children. For a change in position, the child can sit in it with his legs straight out. A card table with the legs cut down makes a good play surface, and contributes to sitting balance.

### Materials for Construction

1. ¾-inch stock
2. Back (*A*), 7½ by 12 inches
3. Base (*B*), 14½ by 18½ inches
4. Sides (*C, D*), 7 by 9 inches each
5. Webbing from sides to point *E* on base

## CLINIC-DESIGNED SITTING INSERT FOR STROLLER

An insert, clinic-designed, can be placed in a stroller to support the completely dependent nonambulatory child (Fig. 1-8*A*). The adapted stroller (Fig. 1-8*B* and *C*) has a number of advantages to provide for the child's comfort and safety:

1. A padded neck rest relieves pressure on the back of the head, helping to minimize extensor thrust.
2. The hip angle is slightly flexed, and the knee angle is approximately a right angle.
3. The feet rest firmly on a baseboard that doubles as a footboard.

4. Straps hold the insert to the stroller.
5. The plastic foam insert within a wooden frame (Fig. 1-8*C*) is covered by a washable cover.
6. A wide plastic foam safety belt is provided for the delicate child who cannot tolerate other types.

## CLINIC-DESIGNED SUPPORTIVE SITTING UNIT

A supportive sitting unit, clinic-designed, is especially suited to the needs of the severely disabled child (Fig. 1-9). It can be used as an isolated unit or as an insert for a larger chair or wheelchair during the feeding period. The design has several outstanding elements:

1. Wings support the child who flails laterally.
2. The backboard has a slight forward pitch (Fig. 1-9*A*) to prevent liquids from dripping onto the child. The position provides for optimal sucking and swallowing.
3. The seat belt (Fig. 1-9*B*) comes from the back lower corners of the unit. Similar to an auto safety belt, it gives security without constricting the chest or stomach. The ends may be attached to the seat with panel cement.
4. A slatted seat insert (Fig. 1-10, patent pending) fits into the unit. It starts flat in the back and is rolled upward at the front to raise the seat under the knees from ½ to 2 inches. This pitches the child's weight back on his thighs and may also help to control extensor thrust.

## BOX SUPPORT

An improvised seat for short-term use for the nursery set is a heavy paper box. The child is seated cross-legged or tailor-fashion inside the box, which gives aid and body support (Fig. 1-11). Quick and safe for short-term use on the lawn, beach, and other recreational areas, it is also helpful for temporary seating while the child gets a snack during "juice time" in the nursery. Additional support can be provided by sandbags to stabilize the sitting position.

## VARIATION OF BOX SUPPORT

A taller box or a plastic wastebasket may also be used. It should be cut down on two sides to provide better vision (Fig. 1-12). Masking tape rolled over the cut edges reinforces them. A firm pillow, against which the child leans, is placed in the tall corner. Facing front, the child looks directly out over the cut corner.

Christine Stephens, OTR, of Montebello State Hospital in Baltimore, Maryland uses heavy, waxed, corrugated boxes used for shipping dressed poultry. She

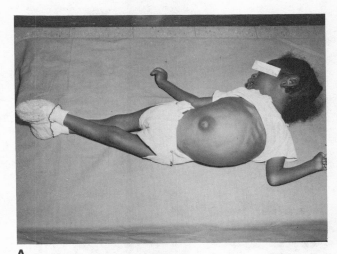

**A**

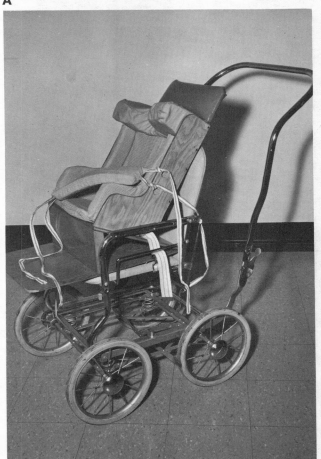

**B**

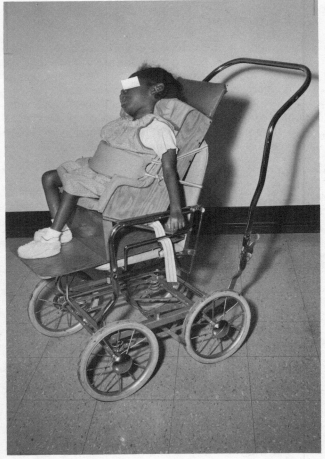

**C**

**FIG. 1-8.** Completely dependent nonambulatory child (*A*) and clinic designed insert in stroller (*B*), in which child can be placed and transferred comfortably and safely (*C*). (Courtesy of A. Slominski, Cerebral Palsy Clinic, Indiana University Medical Center )

advises the use of discarded belts drawn through slits in the sides and base to support the trunk and control the hips and legs of the child. The belts can also be used to strap the seat into a chair or to a dining table leg. Or the seats can be backed into a corner of the room, a living room chair, or the back seat of a car with equal ease and security. A whole box with top can provide both support and play table for a very small child by cutting a triangular piece out of the lid corner to fit the child's chest. A cushion in the bottom corner can raise the child to the desired height for using the arms in extension or flexion in relation to the "table" surface.

## ROCKER

A rocker can be made from a cut-down apple crate (Fig. 1-13). A pillow is used to fill in space and give back support. The child sits cross-legged. The rocker is fun in nursery settings and is useful, as well, for the development of proprioception and for balance training.

## SUPPORT FRAME

A support frame places a child in a position of relaxation, allowing him to move his arms freely and use both hands in activities (Fig. 1-14). With the use of stimulating activities, children have accepted the frame. It lends itself to a moment of free expression, as in finger painting. The frame can be placed close to a sandbox or an inflatable swimming pool where the nonstructure and tactile stimulation of sand or water are very enticing.

The apparatus, compact in its design, is easily stored. Its light weight makes it practical as a piece of loan equipment.

### Construction

The frame is made of ½-inch plywood. The supporting surface and sides are padded with sponge rubber covered with upholstering plastic or Naugahyde.

The size of the frame (Fig. 1-15) was proportioned to the average measurements of a child 3½ to 5 years of age. The overall length, approximately 29 inches, supports the prone body from the superior portion of the sternum to the ankle. This length, as well as the height of the foot end, permits free dorsiflexion and plantar flexion and adds to the comfort of the patient.

The 10-inch width of the bed extends from the ankle to the axilla. The width is reduced to 4 inches for the

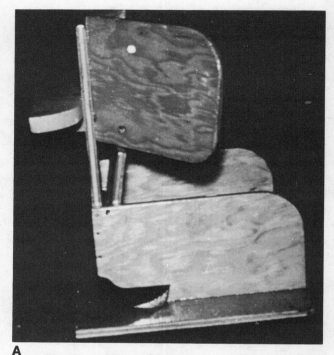

A

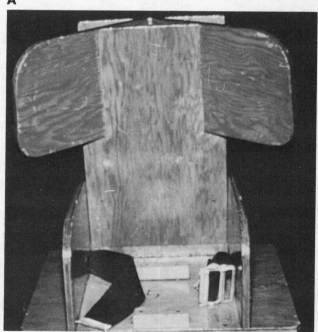

B

FIG. 1-9. Seating insert, clinic-designed, for larger chair or wheelchair. (A) Side view, showing slight forward pitch of backboard. (B) Front view, showing attachment of seat belt at back lower corners. (Courtesy of A. Slominski, Cerebral Palsy Clinic, Indiana University Medical Center)

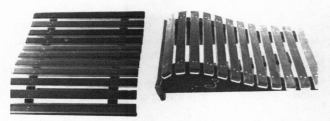

**FIG. 1-10.** Slatted seat insert (patent pending) to fit into special seating unit, to provide upward lift to knees. (Courtesy of A. Slominski, Cerebral Palsy Clinic, Indiana University Medical Center )

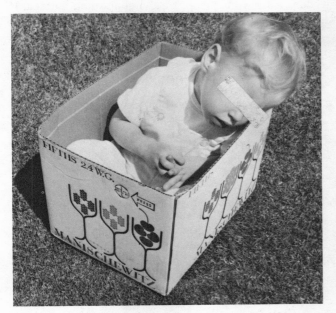

**FIG. 1-11.** Heavy paper box used as seating aid. Child shown needs additional support of sandbags to stabilize his position. (Courtesy of A. Wolfe, University of California Developmental Center, Los Angeles)

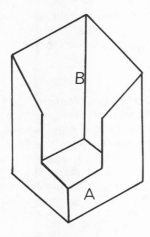

**FIG. 1-12.** Variation of box support, with corner, *A,* cut out to provide better vision. Pillow for additional support can be placed against tall corner, *B.* (Courtesy of A. Wolfe, University of California Developmental Center, Los Angeles)

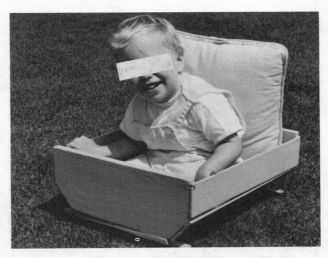

**FIG. 1-13.** Rocker made from apple crate, with pillow for additional support. (Courtesy of P. Holser Buehler)

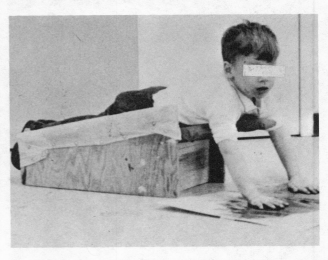

**FIG. 1-14.** Support frame, affording relaxation and free arm movement. (From Yandric, G. G. Support frame for cerebral palsy children. *Amer J Occup Ther 20:*151, 1966. Reproduced with permission)

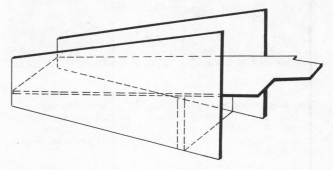

**FIG. 1-15.** Schematic diagram of support frame, showing construction. (From Yandric, G. G. Support frame for cerebral palsy children. *Amer J Occup Ther 20:*151, 1966. Reproduced with permission)

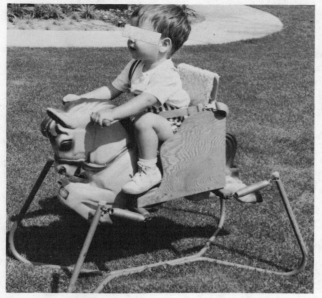

**A**

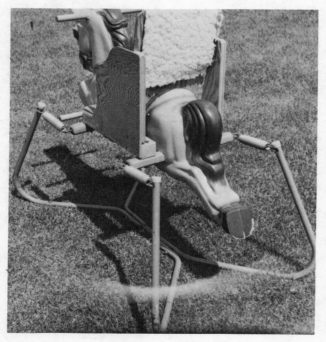

**B**

**FIG. 1-16.** Wooden seat built around body of rocking horse. (*A*) Seat belt holds child in place. (*B*) Curved bottom edge of back fits snugly to body of rocking horse. (Courtesy of A. Johnson, University of California Developmental Center, Los Angeles)

remaining 4 inches of length. This projection provides support to the chest and facilitates voluntary movement at the sternoclavicular, acromioclavicular, and glenohumeral joints. Elevating the head end 8 inches allows gravity to bring the shoulders into flexion and the elbows into full extension.

Frequently, involuntary movements may be present in the lower extremities, inducing awkwardness and fatigue. In an attempt to control this and to prevent the child from falling out, the sides of the frame have been raised 4 inches above the supporting surface. If additional security is needed, a double sandbag may be laid across the gluteal area or straps may be attached to the supporting surface to fasten the child in.

## MODIFIED SEAT FOR ROCKING HORSE

A wooden seat can be built around the body of a rocking horse to permit its use by the child with poor sitting balance (Fig. 1-16). A seat belt should be attached to hold him in place.

### Precaution

Check the seat belt. If it cuts in under the child's rib flare, its position should be changed. The best position for the seat belt in all situations is a slot near the junction of the seat and the back, as with auto safety belts.

## MODIFIED CAPTAIN'S CHAIR

A chair that is less cumbersome than the usual relaxation chair is a captain's chair of small size, remodeled to meet the child's needs (Fig. 1-17). The back and sides give support and security. The chair is useful for preschoolers with short thighs. Most seats are too deep for them, and their feet cannot reach the floor. A seat belt near the hips, similar to an auto safety belt, is the preferred restrainer.

### Remodeling

See directions under Measurements for Special Equipment earlier in this chapter. Get the depth of seat measurement for the child who is to be fitted. Apply this measurement from the back of the chair toward the front, marking it where it ends. Cut away the excess in front of the mark, shaping it in a wide "U" (Fig. 1-17*B*). This will leave some protection at the sides to keep the child's legs from flopping outward.

The height of the chair need not be cut down if a

footrest is used. By making the footrest removable, the chair will be useful for a longer period of time as the child grows.

## COMMERCIAL UTILITY CHAIRS

Several specially made chairs are available. The general precautions for chairs, listed at the beginning of this chapter are to be observed in purchasing equipment, just as they are when building equipment.

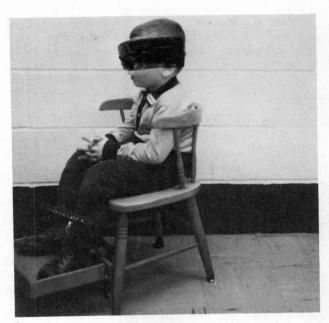

**A**

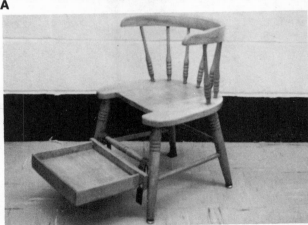

**B**

**FIG. 1-17.** Captain's chair modified to give support and security (*A*). (*B*) With footrest and cut-away seat. (Courtesy of S. Reed, Cooperative Preschool for Children and United Cerebral Palsy of Western New York, Inc.)

### Sources

Besides the sources listed here, catalogs of manufacturers and distributors of school equipment contain various types of sturdy kindergarten chairs.

Adjusta-Chair Co.
J. J. Block
Community Playthings
Fairway King, Inc.
Hausmann Industries, Inc.
Invacare Corp.
J. A. Preston Corp.
J. L. Warren, Inc.
American Hospital Supply

### CHILD'S STANDARD CHAIR PC 4506

The chair (Fig. 1-18) is made of solid hard maple, with steam-bent seat frame, stretcher, and back posts, and with solid wood saddle seat. It comes in natural maple, dark maple, walnut, or mahogany finish. The height of the seat should be specified, in inches, when ordering: 10 or 11; 12 or 13; 14 or 15; 16 or 17; 18 (adult).

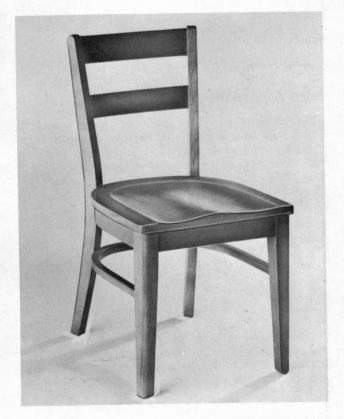

**FIG. 1-18.** Children's standard chair PC 4506. (Copyright 1965 by J. A. Preston Corporation)

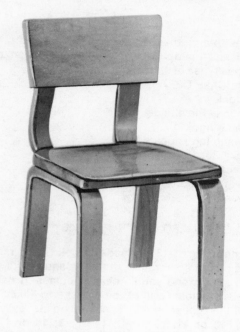

**FIG. 1-19.** Children's "Bentply" chair PC 4507. (Copyright 1965 by J. A. Preston Corporation)

## Source

J. A. Preston Corp.

## CHILDREN'S "BENTPLY" CHAIR PC 4507

This chair (Fig. 1-19) is made of bent plywood, is light weight, and is extremely durable. Except for the 10- and 12-inch chairs, it has a solid saddle seat and back bow. The colors are the same as those of PC 4506. The height of the seat, in inches, should be specified when ordering: 10 to 12; 13 to 14; 15 or 16; 17; 18 (adult).

## Source

J. A. Preston Corp.

## ALL-ADJUSTABLE KINDERGARTEN CHAIR PC 4505

This chair (Fig. 1-20) has a chrome-plated tubular steel frame and molded Fiberglas seat, 12 inches wide and adjustable in depth from 12 inches to 6 inches. Seat color is beige. The nylon-reinforced plastic back, in beige color, is designed so that the back may be

rigid if required. The footboard adjusts from 10½ to 4 inches from the seat. The height of the arms from the floor is 18½ inches. A 58-inch-long strap with instant release hitch may be used as a body or leg strap. This chair is also for athetoid patients. The weight of the chair is 17 pounds.

## Source

J. A. Preston Corp.

## CHAIR TRAY PC 4505T

The all-adjustable kindergarten chair (PC 4505) also comes with a plastic-topped tray with a raised rim, 24 by 24 inches, with a 6- by 9-inch cutout. The weight is 10 pounds.

## Source

J. A. Preston Corp.

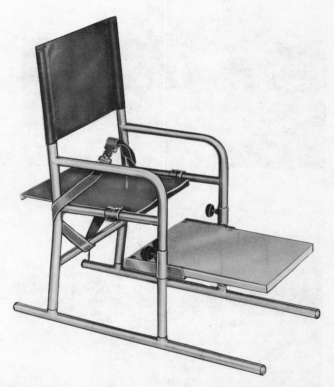

**FIG. 1-20.** All-adjustable kindergarten chair PC 4505, with adjustable height, seat position, and footrest. (Copyright 1965 by J. A. Preston Corporation)

## MODIFIED ALL-ADJUSTABLE KINDERGARTEN CHAIR

A modification of the all-adjustable kindergarten chair is recommended by A. Johnson and A. Wolfe, of the United Cerebral Palsy–Developmental Center at UCLA, as being particularly suitable as a classroom chair for the child who cannot sit in a regular chair (Fig. 1-21). Its greatest advantages are: (1) The adjustable footrest with heel and toe loops and recesses for the feet. This assures the child of foot support at all times. (2) The adjustable seat, which can be moved forward or back to assure proper placement of the child's hips in relation to the back rest. A wedge-shaped cushion helps assure jack-knife position. Another advantage is the sled runners, which make the chair easy to push about and tip-proof.

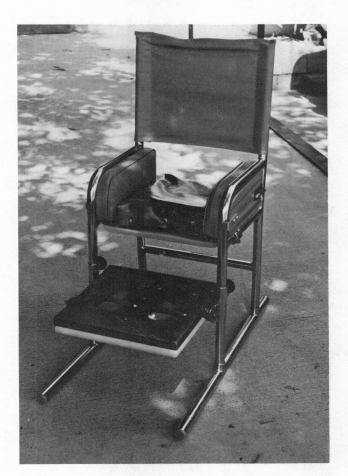

**FIG. 1-21.** Modification of the all-adjustable kindergarten chair (Invacare Corp., Elyria, Ohio)

Side supports of wood padded with foam rubber stay in place in the chair by means of a metal cleat on one end and a sliding bolt lock at the other. They are useful for the child for whom the chair is too wide, and can be removed easily. All modifications were ordered by UCP-UCLA from Invalex, Lodi, Ohio, to meet specified nursery needs.

### Precaution

For children whose feet become caught between the footboard area and the chair seat, lace a piece of canvas between the two front chair legs.

## TOILET EQUIPMENT

### TOILET ADAPTATION

A new sanitary apparatus is the "Closomat Atlantic" (Fig. 1-22). A warm water douche at body temperature and warm air provides hygienic personal cleansing while eliminating the use of hands.

### Source

Spies Trading Co.

### ADJUSTABLE POTTY CHAIR

The seat of this chair is commode type. The height can be adjusted from 11 inches to 16 inches by means of telescoping legs. The arms give limited side support (Fig. 1-23). An extension may be added to the back if necessary. Of intermediate size, the chair is good until the child is large enough for a regular commode chair or toilet.

### Source

Invacare Corp.

### CLINIC-DESIGNED POTTY CHAIR

A clinic-designed potty chair especially for preschool children (Fig. 1-24) has several useful features. The sides extend to the back to prevent tipping (Fig. 1-24*B*). In the back itself is a slot near the top to facilitate lifting and placement of the chair where it is needed. There is a back opening for potty removal. The seatboard, with potty hole, slants downward 6 degrees to the back. A removable tray (Fig. 1-24*C*) eliminates the child's fear of falling and serves as an armrest, thus aiding relaxation.

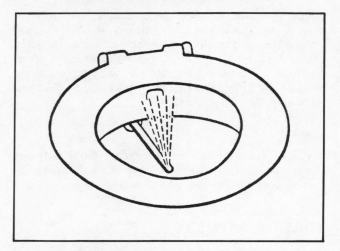

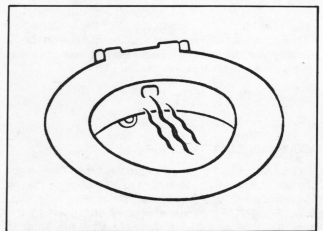

**FIG. 1-22.** Diagram of sanitary apparatus. (Courtesy of Spies Trading Co., Bloomfield, N.J.)

## TOILET ADAPTATIONS FOR NURSERY SCHOOL FACILITIES

Several pointers may be helpful in meeting the toilet needs of children:

1. Equipment should fit the children for size and for self-help activities (Fig. 1-25).
2. Sinks should be low enough for children to reach.
3. Some of the potty chairs should be low enough for the child's feet to reach the floor.
4. Potty chairs designed for taller children may be used by smaller children if they have a box stabilized by a sandbag to hold it at the proper level to be a footrest (Fig. 1-26).
5. A seat belt, from the back, similar to auto safety belts, should be used.

6. A post should be provided on the boys' potty chair, to serve as a deflector (Fig. 1-26), not just a leg spreader.

See also the potty chair combination with stand-in table later in this chapter.

## CLINIC-DESIGNED TOILET TRAINING CHAIR FOR OLDER CHILD

For the nonambulatory, non-toilet-trained teenager (Fig. 1-27A), inserts can be built to fit a chair on wheels (Fig. 1-27B), so that it can be rolled to the bathroom and positioned over the toilet. The chair has a slightly flexed seat, a slightly flexed footrest, and a slanted backboard to accommodate fetal back curve. A seat belt is provided for security. A tray hooks onto the wooden insert to aid optimal positioning (Fig. 1-27C).

The child was toilet-trained at the clinic in two weeks' time by the Clock Method.

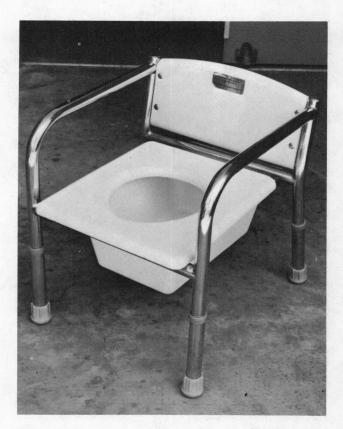

**FIG. 1-23.** Adjustable potty chair suitable for small child. (Invacare Corp., Elyria, Ohio)

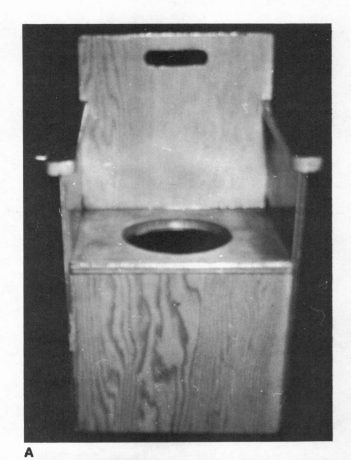

**A**

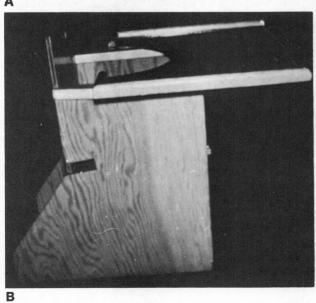

**B**

FIG. 1-24. Clinic-designed potty chair. (*A*) Front view. (*B*) Extension of sides to the back to prevent tipping. (*C*) Tray eliminates fear of falling. (Courtesy of A. Slominski, Cerebral Palsy Clinic, Indiana University Medical Center)

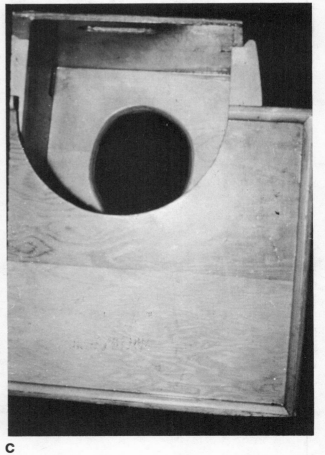

**C**

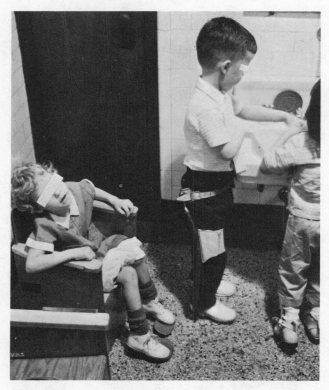

**FIG. 1-25.** Equipment adapted to size of children, with sinks low enough for self-help and potty chairs low enough for feet to reach floor. (Courtesy of A. Slominski, Cerebral Palsy Clinic, Indiana University Medical Center; reproduced with permission)

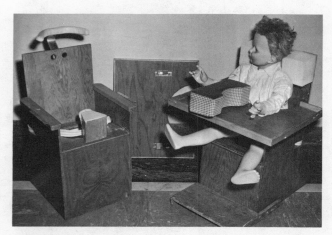

**FIG. 1-26.** Potty chair stabilized by sandbags; box provides footrest. (Courtesy A. Slominski, Cerebral Palsy Clinic, Indiana University Medical Center. Reproduced with permission)

## RELAXATION CHAIRS

Before purchasing or constructing special chairs, give due consideration to the use of adaptations of regular chairs and wheelchairs. Inserts, seat belts, footrests, and cut-out trays and tables to stabilize the child often convert wheelchairs into useful supportive seating and give the added advantage of mobility. If a relaxation chair is chosen, several precautions should be taken.

### Precautions

1. Always put a relaxation chair on wheels to facilitate a change of environment.
2. Always use a tray or cut-out table on which the child's arms may rest and which will stabilize his position.
3. If extensor thrust is augmented by a right-angle footrest and by the child's head hitting the back of the chair, put sandbags under his feet to dorsiflex and try attaching a neck pillow or suitable substitute.
4. A tray is usually sufficient support, but if not, use a safety belt placed at the same angle recommended for auto safety belts. Diagonal belts, as found in foreign cars or similar to shoulder belts, are preferable to chest binders. Never let the belt cut under the rib cage or bind the stomach area.

## RELAXATION CHAIR PC 4503

This sturdily constructed chair (Fig. 1-28) reclines easily to a 63-degree angle. The footrest is adjustable for height by sliding it into the appropriate groove. The 22- by 24-inch tray is detachable and has a rim around it; the tray top is stainproof heavy plastic. The seat is 12 inches wide by 12 inches deep. Overall measurements are: length, 24 inches; width, 15 inches; height, 36 inches. The chair comes in an attractive natural wood finish and has four ball-bearing casters.

### Source

J. A. Preston Corp.

## RELAXATION CHAIR PC 4504

A popular economy-priced chair (Fig. 1-29), this one reclines at various angles up to 65 degrees. The footrest is adjustable in height to accommodate the height of the child. The seat measures 12 inches wide by

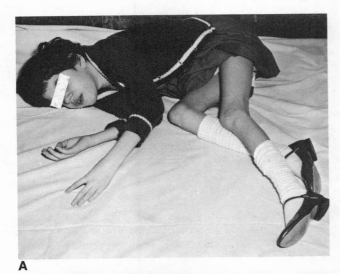

**A**

FIG. 1-27. For nonambulatory, non-toilet-trained teenager (*A*), clinic-designed insert for chair on wheels (*B*) that can be rolled to bathroom (*C*). (Courtesy of A. Slominski, Cerebral Palsy Clinic, Indiana University Medical Center)

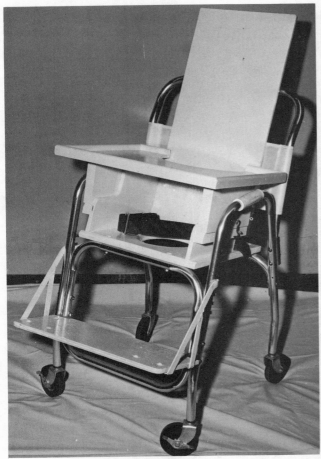

**B**

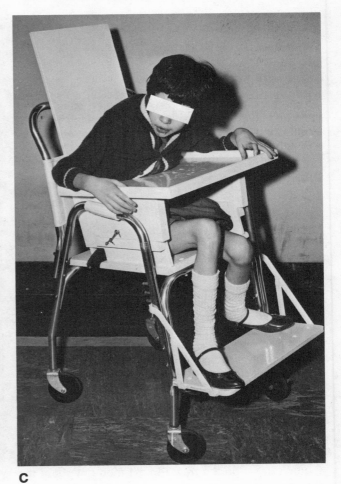

**C**

11½ inches deep. The chair is constructed of plywood with an attractive pale green lacquer finish.

Also available for this chair are a set of blocks (PC 4504B) to narrow the seat by 1½ inches; a set of 2-inch ball-bearing casters (PC 4504C); and a detachable tray (PC 4504D) with a scratch-resistant plastic top, 24 by 24 inches, with a raised ledge.

### Source

J. A. Preston Corp.

### RELAXATION CHAIR WITH TRAY PC 4501MA

This chair is an institutional model with a metal base (Fig. 1-30). The standard size of the chair is 46 inches in overall height, with a 13½ by 13½-inch seat, and a 24- by 30-inch tray with an 8- by 12-inch cutout.

### Source

J. A. Preston Corp.

### HEAVY-DUTY CHAIR

This relaxation chair (Fig. 1-31) may be constructed. However, before undertaking the task, weigh carefully whether it will have any advantage over a wheelchair with adjustments.

### Construction

1. The suggested material for this chair is ¾-inch plywood.
2. Back piece (*A*). Measure from top of shoulder to base of backbone.
3. Seat (*B*). Measure from back to 1 inch before the bend of the knee.
4. Distance from knee to footrest (*C*). Measure from the bend of the knee to the sole of the foot. If necessary, the foot angle may be adjusted with a sandbag or a wedge block made to order.
5. Width of chair (*D*). Measure across hips at back when child is sitting. Add 1 inch to each side, never narrower. If seat is made wider, inserts may be added for supportive sitting or for adjustment to different children.
6. Lapboard (*E*). Cut board in a semicircle to fit child. The size of the board depends on child's reach with his arms. The height of the lapboard should allow the child's arms, when bent at the elbow, to rest comfortably on the tray. Put a 1-inch rim about the board.

7. Wheels (*F*). These should be large enough to roll easily over doorsills, allowing for change of location. Some method of braking wheels should be considered for inclines.
8. Seat belt (*G*). If used, seat belt should be at the position of auto safety belts. Use wide webbing, not tight narrow leather.
9. Cutout in base (*H*). A cut-out section on the back edge of the base will enable person pushing the chair to get near to it. The size of the base depends on the overall size of the chair.

### ADJUSTABLE CHAIR

Before constructing this chair (Fig. 1-32), decide what advantage this type of chair would have over a wheelchair with clinic-designed inserts made to meet the patient's needs.

**FIG. 1-28.** Relaxation chair PC 4503. (Copyright by J. A. Preston Corporation)

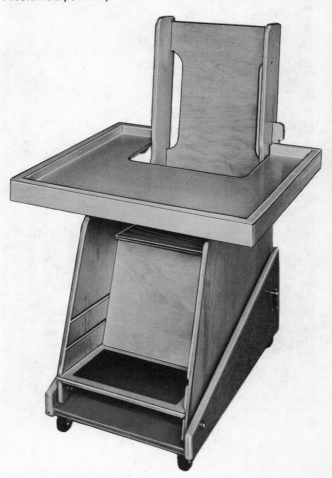

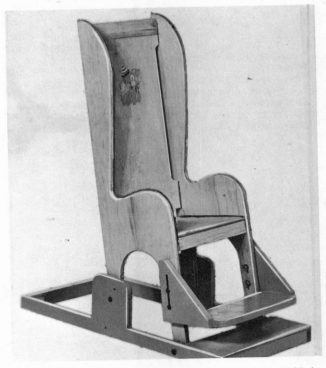

**FIG. 1-29.** Relaxation chair PC 4504. (Copyright 1965 by J. A. Preston Corporation)

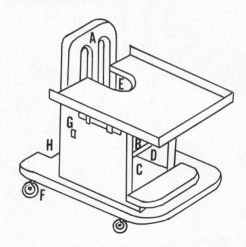

**FIG. 1-31.** Heavy duty chair that may be constructed. *A,* back piece; *B,* seat; *C,* distance from seat to footrest; *D,* width of chair; *E,* lapboard; *F,* wheels; *G,* slot for seat belt; *H,* base of chair, with cutout. (Courtesy of Cerebral Palsy Unit New York State Rehabilitation Hospital, West Haverstraw, N.Y.)

**Construction Pointers**

1. All stock should be ½-inch thick.
2. Unspecified radii are 1 inch.
3. All wing nuts, bolts, and nuts are ⅜ inch in diameter. Holes (*D*) should be large enough to accommodate this size bolt.

**Precautions**

1. Never use the tip-back position for feeding.
2. Never use the chair without a tray cut to fit the child, unless the chair is at a table of suitable height for good posture.
3. Put wheels on the chair that are large enough to roll over doorsills; provide some method to brake the chair.
4. Put seat belts, if they are needed, at the position of auto safety belts. Make these of wide webbing, not narrow leather.
5. Never make the chair too narrow or too deep; adjust with inserts if necessary.
6. Use a wedge, made to fit, on the footrest, if necessary to achieve proper angle of the feet.

GAD-ABOUT CHAIR WITH ADJUSTABLE TABLE

A handy gad-about chair (Fig. 1-33) can be constructed. Not visible in the photographs are the slots for insertion of an auto type seat belt at hip level.

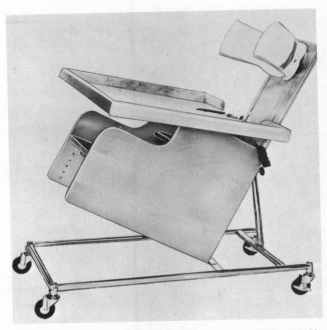

**FIG. 1-30.** Relaxation chair-tray combination PC 4501MA. (Copyright by J. A. Preston Corporation)

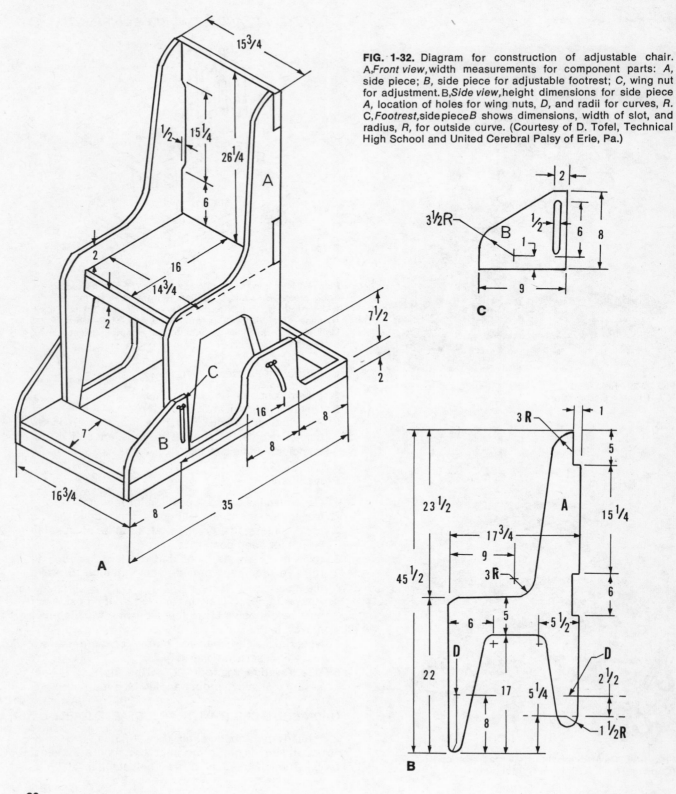

**FIG. 1-32.** Diagram for construction of adjustable chair. A, *Front view,* width measurements for component parts: *A,* side piece; *B,* side piece for adjustable footrest; *C,* wing nut for adjustment. B, *Side view,* height dimensions for side piece *A,* location of holes for wing nuts, *D,* and radii for curves, *R.* C, *Footrest,* side piece *B* shows dimensions, width of slot, and radius, *R,* for outside curve. (Courtesy of D. Tofel, Technical High School and United Cerebral Palsy of Erie, Pa.)

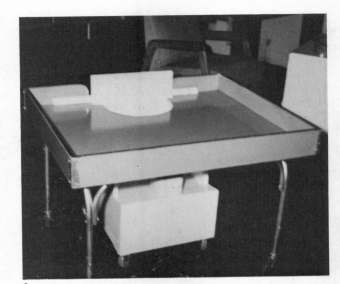

A

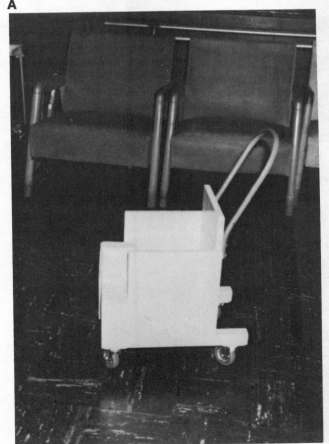

B

**FIG. 1-33.** Gad-about chair. (*A*) Chair with adjustable table in place. (*B*) Side view without table. (*C*) Rear view with table in place. (*D*) Table with cutouts to fit child and to hold dish and cup in place. (Courtesy of G. Fullan, Spastic Aid of Alabama, Inc., Birmingham)

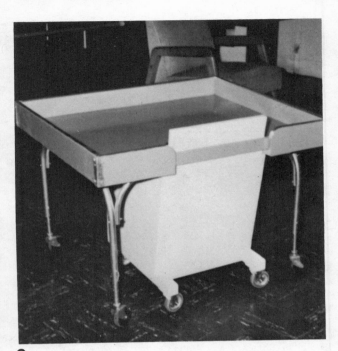

C

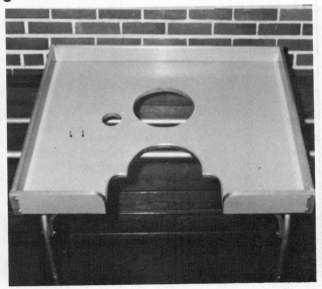

D

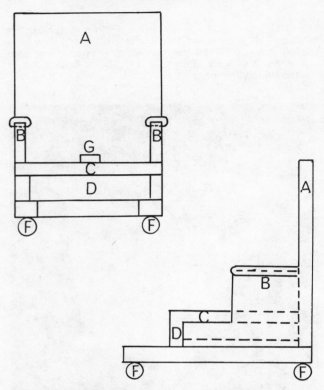

**FIG. 1-34.** Diagram of front and side views for construction of gad-about chair. *A,* back; *B,* side arms; *C,* seat; *D,* front piece; *E,* base; *F,* casters; *G,* slot for seat belt. (Courtesy of G. Fullan, Spastic Aid of Alabama, Inc., Birmingham)

## Construction

Figures 1-34 and 1-35 show front and side views of the chair and the dimensions of the various parts.
1. The back height can be made to suit the rider or the pusher.
2. Use ¾-inch weatherproof plywood for all chair parts.
3. Use 2- by 2-inch wood for base frame.
4. Cover chair arms with sponge rubber, 1 inch thick, and plastic upholstering material for comfort and cleanliness.
5. Use casters large enough for easy mobility (Colson No. 37253 or equivalent or 3-inch rubber tires that can swivel).

## Precaution

Use weatherproof wood and round all corners and edges.

## CUT-OUT TABLES

### CUT-OUT TABLE PC 4514D

This table (Fig. 1-36) can be used for sitting or standing, since the height is readily adjustable from 21 inches to 33 inches. The offset legs afford greater stability when the child is standing, as he is practically in the center of the table. The cut-out area measures 7 by 10 inches or can be made to specifications. The door can be swung either down or out. Table top is 24 by 30 inches, with a 2-inch rim around it, and is covered with a gray linen mar-resistant plastic.

### Source

J. A. Preston Corp.

### CUT-OUT TABLE PC 4515A

The height of this table (Fig. 1-37) is also adjustable, from 22 to 35 inches. The 24- by 24-inch top is covered with scratch-resistant plastic and has a ledge around it. The table comes in a natural wood finish with chrome trim.

### Source

J. A. Preston Corp.

### CLINIC TYPE CUT-OUT TABLE PC 4515B

This table is similar to PC 4515A, with height adjustable from 22 to 35 inches, but the top is larger, 24 by 36 inches, covered with plastic. A ledge surrounds the top. Finish is natural wood, with chrome trim.

### Source

J. A. Preston Corp.

### FOUR-PLACE CUT-OUT TABLE PC 4516A

The functional kidney-shaped construction of this table (Fig. 1-38) allows plenty of room for each child. The top is 29 inches wide and 96 inches long, and is covered with a gray linen mar-resistant plastic, bonded to ¾-inch plywood, metal trimmed. All corners are carefully rounded. The height is 24 inches. Cut-out sections vary in size: one, 6 by 9 inches; one, 8 by 12 inches; and two, 7 by 10 inches (other sizes

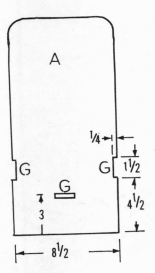

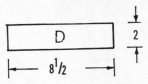

**FIG. 1-35.** Diagram of parts, for construction of gad-about chair, giving dimensions. *A*, back with slots *G* for seat belt; *B*, side arms; *C*, seat; *D*, front piece; *E*, base (dotted line shows inside cutout); *F*, depth of base and width for positioning of side arms at rear of base. (Courtesy of G. Fullan, Spastic Aid of Alabama, Inc., Birmingham)

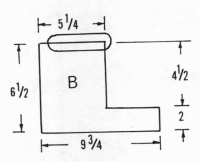

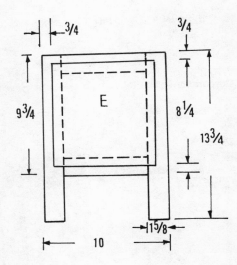

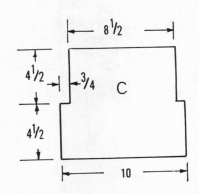

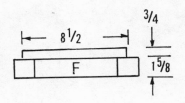

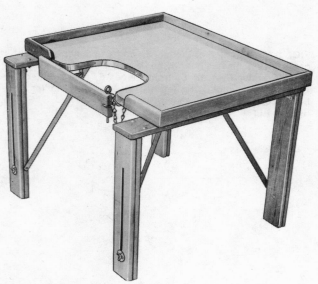

**FIG. 1-36.** Cut-out table PC 4514D. (Copyright 1965 by J. A. Preston Corporation)

**FIG. 1-37.** Cut-out table PC 4515A. (Copyright 1965 by J. A. Preston Corporation)

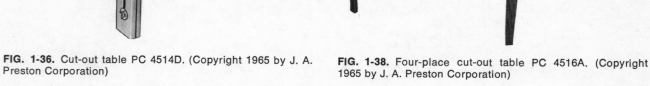

**FIG. 1-38.** Four-place cut-out table PC 4516A. (Copyright 1965 by J. A. Preston Corporation)

**FIG. 1-39.** Diagram for construction of adjustable cut-out table. (Courtesy of Cerebral Palsy Unit, New York State Rehabilitation Hospital, West Haverstraw, N.Y.)

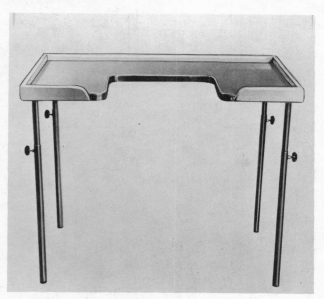

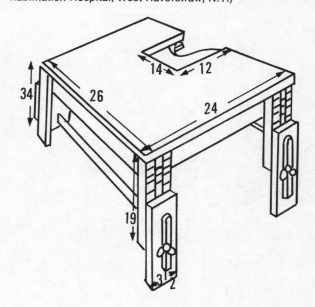

are available at no additional charge). Legs are steam-bent plywood in modern design.

A similar table (PC 4516W) is available without the cutouts. It seats up to six children.

## Source

J. A. Preston Corp.

## ADJUSTABLE CUT-OUT TABLE

A cut-out table that is adjustable in height can be constructed (Fig. 1-39).

## Construction

1. Use ¾-inch plywood.
2. Make legs in two parts, slotted so that bolts and wing nuts may be used to adjust the height of the table. Height with legs extended is 34 inches.
3. Make variety of inserts for the cutout, to meet the needs and contours of individual children.
4. Secure two webbed straps to the table on each side of the cut-out section. They can be closed by means of an adjustable buckle to support those children needing extra stability.

**FIG. 1-40.** Clinic type stand-in table PC 4513B. (Copyright 1965 by J. A. Preston Corporation)

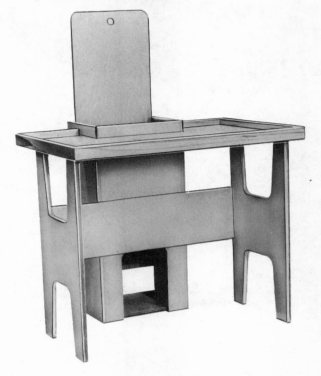

## STAND-IN TABLES

### CLINIC TYPE STAND-IN TABLE PC 4513B

The stand-in box of this table (Fig. 1-40) is 14 inches wide and 10 inches deep. A special back and head support, included with the table, can be inserted in two positions to reduce the depth of the box to 9 inches or 8 inches. The foot platform adjusts instantly. The 24- by 36-inch top is covered with scratch-resistant plastic.

## Source

J. A. Preston Corp.

### CLINIC TYPE STAND-IN TABLE PC 4513C

This unit (Fig. 1-41) is sturdily constructed and is placed on a wide base to prevent tipping. The box is made of attractive ¾-inch birch plywood. The foot platform is rubber-covered and adjusts from 22 inches to 32 inches from the top. Table height is 33½ inches. The top measures 30 by 24 inches and is covered with gray linen mar-resistant plastic. The edges are raised. The cut-out area is 7 by 10 inches, but other sizes— 6 by 9 inches, 8 by 12 inches, and 9 by 15 inches— are available at no extra cost.

## Source

J. A. Preston Corp.

## Precautions

1. Use two locks or hook locks to prevent the door of the stand-in box from opening.
2. Use air holes or screening to keep the box cool in hot weather.

### GROUP TYPE STAND-IN TABLES

Several types of stand-in tables for groups are also available (Figs. 1-42 and 1-43).

## Sources

J. J. Block
G. E. Miller, Inc.
J. A. Preston Corp.

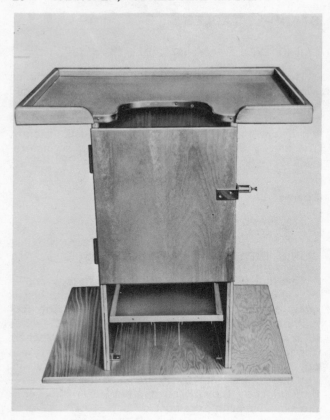

**FIG. 1-41.** Clinic type stand-in table PC 4513C. (Copyright 1965 by J. A. Preston Corporation)

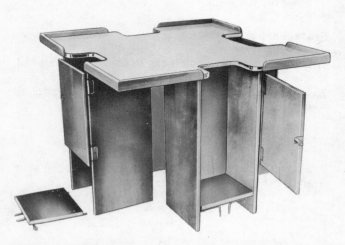

**FIG. 1-42.** Group type stand-in table to accommodate four children PC 5417. (Copyright 1965 by J. A. Preston Corporation)

## STAND-IN TABLE TYPE I

This table (Fig. 1-44) can be constructed for individuals with fair standing ability and trunk control. Although the height of the table is stationary, the child can be raised via the footboard since less support is required. There is also an adjustable leg spreader for those who "scissor."

### Construction

1. Footboard (*A*). Adjustable by placement at several levels.
2. Leg spreader (*B*). Slotted track makes height adjustable to level of footboard. A butterfly screw in front and metal plate in back hold the spreader in place.
3. Gate (*C*). This can be padded, if necessary. Or a wide web belt may be used instead.
4. Cut-out area of table top (*D*). Line this with metal.

## STAND-IN TABLE TYPE II

This is an adjustable table, clinic-designed, with chair and potty chair adaptations (Fig. 1-45). The arm rests slide up or down in slots. The table hooks onto the arm rests, and thus both table top and arm rests

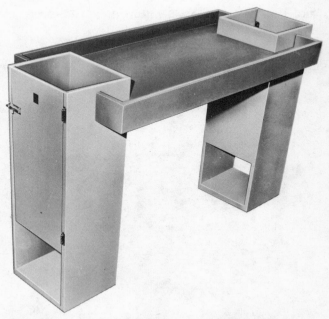

**FIG. 1-43.** Stand-in table to accommodate two children, PC 4521. (Copyright 1965 by J. A. Preston Corporation)

are adapted to the size of the child. A safety belt is located in the area of the hip joint. There is a feet divider on the footboard, and wheels at the four corners of the base. A slot at the top of the back provides a handle for an adult to move the table.

With the armrests down in the slots, the table is converted to a chair or potty chair by the use of inserts (Fig. 1-45*B*). The table may be attached with the child in sitting position.

### Construction

Modification of Stand-In Table Type I.

## STAND-IN TABLE TYPE III

This adjustable table (Fig. 1-46) has a body box and runners that extend beyond the table's back legs to ensure greater stability.

### Materials and Measurements

Dimensions given are for a child 2 to 4 years of age. For a larger child, the measurements would need to be increased proportionately.

1. Use plywood for the box. For height see Construction. Width and depth are 10½ by 10½ inches. Door is approximately 9 by 16 inches. Attach bolts to door, one 4 inches from top, one 12 inches from top.
2. Use 5-ply plywood for the runners. Two side pieces are needed, 2 by 25 inches each. The front strip is 2 by 30 inches. The back strips should be long enough to reach the enclosure, depending on the size of the box.
3. Use 5-ply plywood for the legs.
4. For table top, use plywood or Masonite, 16½ by 28½ inches, with cutout for the box. Cover with linoleum, if desired.

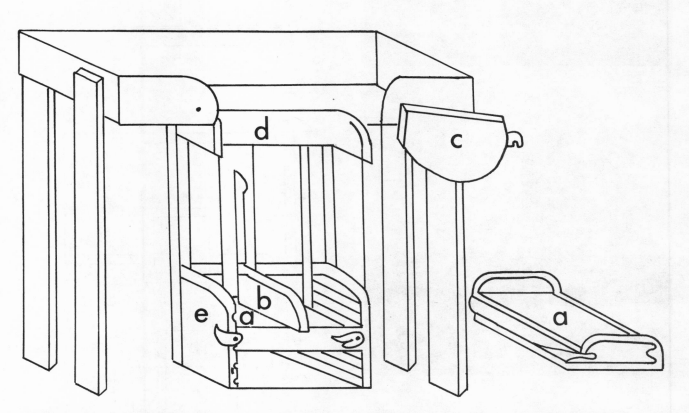

**FIG. 1-44.** Diagram for construction of stand-in table, Type I. *A,* adjustable footboard; *B,* leg spreader, adjustable in height by movement in slotted track; *C,* gate; *D,* cut; *E,* wooden base with grooved sides to accommodate footboard. (Courtesy of Cerebral Palsy Unit, New York State Rehabilitation Hospital, West Haverstraw, N.Y.)

**FIG. 1-45.** Stand-in table Type II. (*A*) Height of table is adjustable. (*B*) Adjusted as potty chair by moving armrests down in slots. (Courtesy of A. Slominski, Cerebral Palsy Clinic, Indiana University Medical Center)

**FIG. 1-46.** Diagram for construction of stand-in table Type III. Side view shows extended runners to ensure stability. Top view gives dimensions for width and depth. Back view gives height dimensions and shows insertion of blocks that form footboard. (Courtesy of Association for Aid of Crippled Children, New York)

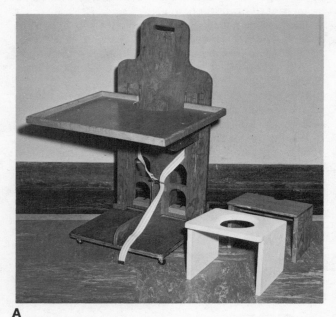

A

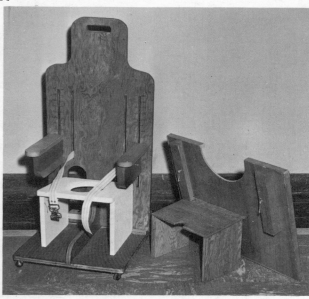

B

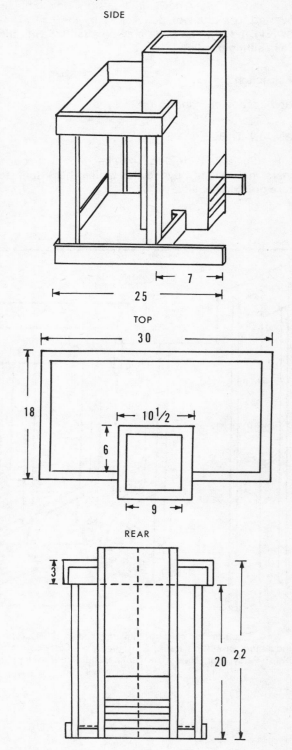

5. Use plywood or Masonite for the rim. The front is 3 by 30 inches; sides, 3 by 18 inches each; back (two pieces), 3 by 9½ inches (or adjusted to size of box).
6. Make blocks of 5-ply plywood, 7¾ inches by 9 inches. Placed in the box, these adjust height.

## Construction

The overall height of the body box should be from a point about 2 to 3 inches below the child's armpits to his feet, plus the thickness of three or four 5-ply plywood blocks on which the child will stand. The blocks must not come up as high as the bottom of the door, or the child's feet cannot be watched to make sure they are in a good weight-bearing position. (These blocks are removed one at a time as the child grows.)

The body box should be inset in the table top for about two-thirds of its depth. The top of the table should come to a height about 4 inches lower than the top of the body box. The 1¼-inch rim around the table prevents toys from being knocked off.

For security, the door is latched with two bolts, one near the top and one near the bottom.

The table legs are secured firmly to the rim around the table top, and a framework is attached to the legs at the floor. The two side pieces of this framework constitute runners extending 7 inches beyond the back legs to prevent the table from tipping backwards. The frame is closed in at the rear and is attached to the body box with an additional 2½-inch piece of plywood.

## Precautions

1. Drill enough holes in the back door to allow air to circulate within the "chimney."
2. Do not allow children to develop the habit of slumping against the body box.

## STAND-IN TABLE TYPE IV

Another type of stand-in table features an extended platform base for stability and slots on the sides of the body box for insertion of the table top (Fig. 1-47).

## Construction

1. Use ½-inch plywood unless otherwise noted.
2. Trim (A), ¾-inch white pine stock.
3. Drill two holes (B), 9/32-inch diameter.
4. Door (C), ¾-inch plywood.
5. Slide bolt (D), 2 inches.

6. Shelving strips (E) for footstand, 8 pieces of ½-inch square white pine, spaced 1 inch apart, 4 to each side.
7. Base (F). Plywood, 24 by 24 inches.
8. Formica (G) for table top.
9. Table top (H). Plywood under Formica, 19½ by 18 inches (see cut-away view, Figure 1-47, *center right,* for cutout).
10. Rim for table top (I). Use ½- by 2-inch white pine stock, one piece 28 inches long, two pieces 19½ inches long.
11. Table slide strips (J). Use 1½-inch square white pine stock, two pieces, 12 inches long.
12. Foam rubber pad (K), ½ inch thick, is optional.
13. Naugahyde (L) to cover pad is optional.
14. Footstand with feet divider (Fig. 1-47, *upper right*) is optional.
15. Casters may be added for mobility.
16. Door hinges, 2-inch size.

## SEAT BELTS AND SAFETY SUPPORTS

A minimal amount of support necessary to improve posture and to prevent a youngster from falling out of his seat should be used. The postural support should be lessened as the child develops control. In positioning safety supports in chairs, wheelchairs, and cars, the two positions used in auto safety belts are most useful:

1. Firmly fastened under the back edge of the seat, crossing over the wearer between the upper thigh and pelvic area. In this position, the belt holds the hips back and firmly in place. This has the added advantage of causing the individual to sit back and rest his weight over his buttocks rather than on the lower spine.
2. Diagonally fastened, from behind one shoulder to the opposite hip bone. The belt is fastened at the approximate junction of the seat and the back of the chair, wheelchair, or auto seat. This is the position of the safety belts of many foreign cars and is similar to the shoulder belts in American cars.

### Materials for Safety Supports

Materials for safety supports and seat belts should be chosen to prevent chafing and, therefore, should not wrinkle or narrow when stretched.

Nylon or cotton webbing is porous, yet firm.

Width depends on the size of the individual. Generally it should not be less than 1½ inches, with the possible exception of tiny children, for whom a 1-inch width may be indicated to avoid chafing. Scout or

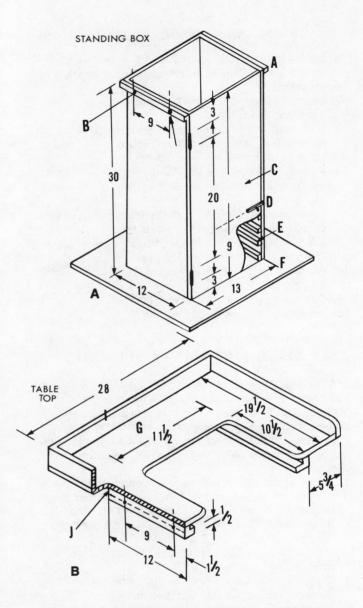

**FIG. 1-47.** Diagram for construction of stand-in table Type IV. *A,* stand-in box, showing location of trim, *A;* position of holes, *B;* for attachment of table; dimensions of door, *C;* position of bolt, *D;* shelving strips for footstand, *E;* and base, *F. B,* cut-away view of table top, with Formica, *G,* applied to table top, *H;* rim, *I;* table slide strips, *J;* pad for inside of box, *K;* and cover for pad, *L. C,* footstand. *D,* table top dimensions, *G,* and slide pieces. (Courtesy of Association for Aid of Crippled Children)

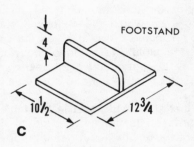

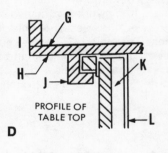

army belts, with their flat buckles, can often be used on young children's equipment as improvised seat belts.

If padding is needed to prevent or correct any mild chafing, cover foam rubber of desired thickness with plastic sheeting that may be sewed or glued to underside of pressure area. Shift the position of the belt or buckle when indicated.

**Precautions**

1. If a child's condition is so serious as to require an actual restraint, it should be medically prescribed.

2. Make a periodic check of every support that is used, to be sure that it does *not* impede circulation, interfere with breathing, or rub the skin at any point.

### AUTOMOBILE RIDING SUPPORT PC 4548A

This support (Fig. 1-48) prevents any tendency of the patient to fall forward or to either side during automobile travel, and is especially useful for young children. The support consists of a stainless steel spring clip and elastic shoulder straps. The clip attaches over the backrest of the car; no permanent

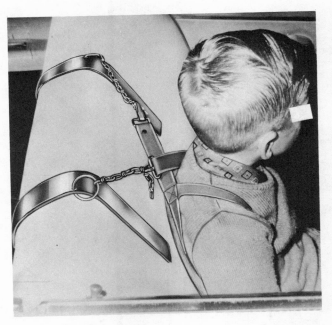

**FIG. 1-48.** Automobile riding support PC 4548A. (Copyright 1965 by J. A. Preston Corporation)

**FIG. 1-49.** Vest for trunk support. Ties at shoulder, *A,* and at underarm, *B.* Loops at waist, *C,* for safety belt. (Courtesy of Warren G. Murray Children's Center, Centralia, Ill.)

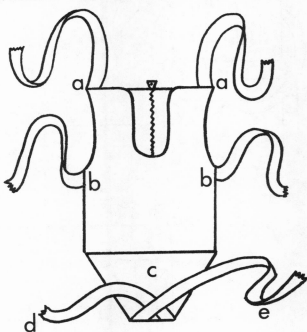

installation is required. The support is designed for patients between 30 and 80 pounds in weight, who are minimally disabled.

**Source**

J. A. Preston Corp.

## VEST FOR TRUNK SUPPORT— ONLY TO BE WORN OVER CLOTHING

A vest can be made to give minimal trunk support (Fig. 1-49) with ties to chair or wheelchair.
1. Ties sewn into shoulder seam at A
2. Ties sewn into side seam at underarm, B
3. The back is elongated so child sits on C and the ties D&E come up between the thighs, with D crossing over right groin and E crossing over left groin to be tied at lower back of chair where seat of chair meets the back. Tie D&E loose enough to allow some free play of legs.

PRECAUTIONS: Cord should never be used for ties; ties should not be narrower than 1-inch webbing.

Article should not be used for anyone whose breathing pattern may be restricted by it, or whose motions cause any of the ties to leave the slightest mark on the skin of the wearer. Inspect frequently.

**Source**

Home made after design used in several clinics

### SAFETY SEAT BELTS

Several types of safety seat belts may be bought or improvised (Fig. 1-50). See also the section on Wheelchair Safety Belts and Supports in Chapter 3.

A belt designed on the principle of the auto safety belt (Fig. 1-51*A*) is placed low at the junction of the trunk and legs.

A belt can be improvised from sheeting strips (Fig. 1-51*B*). Start with a loop around the back chair post, bringing the strips forward. The child sits on the strips, which are then looped over each leg and tied behind the chair.

Another belt (Fig. 1-51*C*) designed on the auto safety belt principle comes over one shoulder and diagonally across to the opposite hip.

A belt for the legs (Fig. 1-51*D*) is fastened at the center of the forward edge of the seat and buckles at the rear of the seat on each side at the hip with webbing buckles, holding the legs separately and firmly.

## CAR SEAT

For the moderately disabled child, a special seat insert (Fig. 1-52) will support him safely and comfortably.

1. A hinge hooks the side pieces to the bottom piece of the wooden seat, allowing the sides to swing down.
2. The car's safety belt comes from behind and over the child, locking both the child and the seat insert to the auto seat (Fig. 1-52*A*).
3. The angle of the back piece gives a slight backward tilt.
4. A wing-shaped neck protector is padded.
5. The side pieces of the insert swing up (Fig. 1-52*B*).
6. A table locks on the side and back (Fig. 1-52*B*), ensuring stability and safety while the child sits relaxed.
7. A box selected for proper size as a footrest may also hold toys for the trip.

## TOP GUARD

A crash-tested commercial product is the Top Guard, which consists of a 5½-pound, hollow, molded polyethylene shield. A removable pad is placed on the inner side of the shield. It is fastened across the child with the auto safety seat belt. The guard is designed for children under 50 pounds.

**Source**

Ford Motor Co.

**FIG. 1-50.** Safety belt attached to chair. (Courtesy of A. Slominski, Cerebral Palsy Clinic, Indiana University Medical Center )

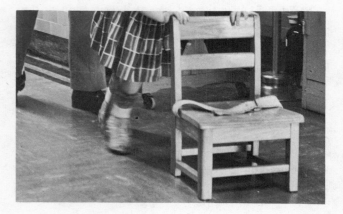

**FIG. 1-51.** Safety belts of various types. (*A*) Like auto safety belt, placed low at junction of trunk and legs. (*B*) Improvised from sheeting strips. (*C*) Diagonal, over shoulder to opposite hip, like auto shoulder belt. (*D*) Webbing attached to chair and buckling at hips.

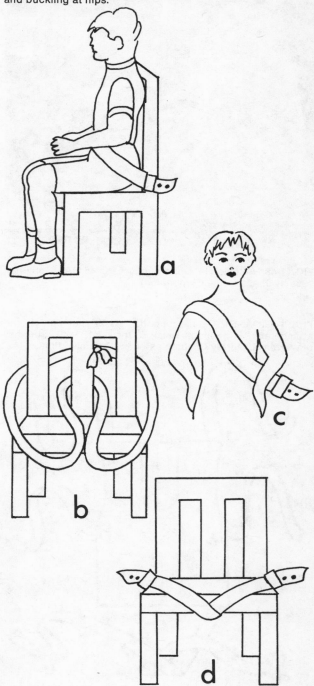

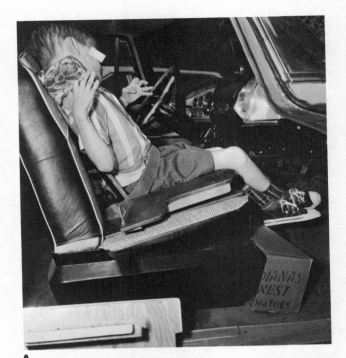

A

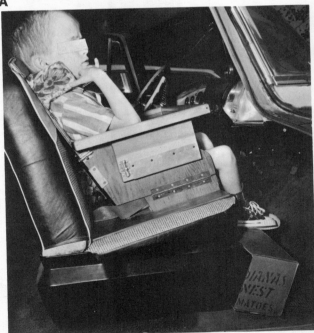

B

**FIG. 1-52.** Car seat insert, open (*A*) and closed (*B*). (Courtesy of A. Slominski, Cerebral Palsy Clinic, Indiana University Medical Center)

# REFERENCES

### Measurements

Dreyfuss, H. *The Measure of Man; Human Factors in Design.* New York, Whitney Publications, Inc., 1959.

*How to Measure the Cerebral Palsied Patient for a Special Chair or Table,* United Cerebral Palsy Association of New York State, 1969.

Morgan, C. *Human Engineering Guide to Equipment Design.* New York, McGraw-Hill, 1963.

Woodson, W., Conover, D. *Human Engineering Guide for Equipment Designers.* Los Angeles, Univ. California Press, 1964.

### Support Frame

Yandric, G. G. "Support frame for cerebral palsy children," Am J Occup Ther 20: 151, 1966.

### Toilet Adaptations for Nursery School Facilities

Bensberg, G. J., ed. *Teaching the Mentally Retarded: A Handbook for Ward Personnel.* Atlanta, Southern Regional Education Board, 1966.

Philips, C. "Devices useful for teaching," J Am Phys Ther, 42:6, 408–409, Ju 1962.

# 2
# Walking Aids

A number of aids have been developed to assist the child in learning to move about on his own. Several good commercially designed products are available, but there are also aids which can be improvised or constructed.

## CREEPERS AND CRAWLERS

### PILLOW CREEPER

A pillow, thick enough for comfort but not so large that the small child's hands and feet cannot reach the floor, is useful when the child learns to creep (Fig. 2-1). If arm and/or leg support is needed, to keep the limb extended, a magazine may be tied around the limb with a wide band tied in a bow.

### BARREL

An older child can be helped to develop gross motor skills by rolling back and forth over a barrel, while supported by an adult (Fig. 2-2). An alternative to the barrel is a large, firm beach ball.

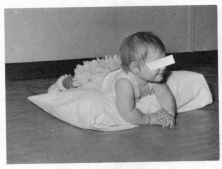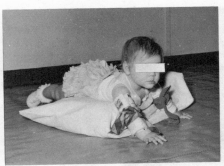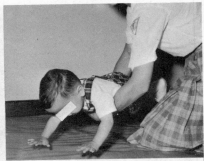

**FIG. 2-1.** Pillow supporting small child learning to creep. Magazines tied around her arms with bows help her to extend her arms. (From Denhoff, E., and Langdon, M., eds. Cerebral dysfunction: A treatment program for young children. *Clin Pediat 5*:332, 1966. Reproduced with permission)

## CLINIC-DESIGNED CREEPER

A creeper has been clinically designed for hand use without leg use (Fig. 2-3). For the child's safety, the creeper incorporates several features:

1. The child's hands are well in front of the wheels so that he cannot roll onto them.
2. The wheels are well under the edges of the board.
3. The board is narrow since the child is not in a cast.
4. The legs are held firmly by wide straps that do not cut, at the knees and ankles and below the buttocks.

## SCOOT-A-BOUT PROPELLED BY ARM ACTION

A creeper that may be used by a child in a cast but is also suitable for other children can be easily constructed at small expense. For the child in a cast (Fig. 2-4), the legs are in a spread-eagle position. Other children should be placed in the most comfortable and functional positions.

**Precaution**

Check the child periodically for pressure points.

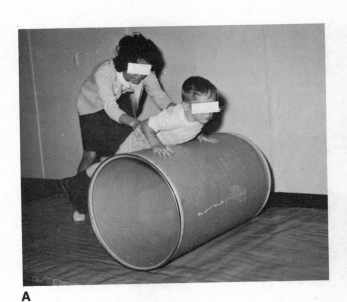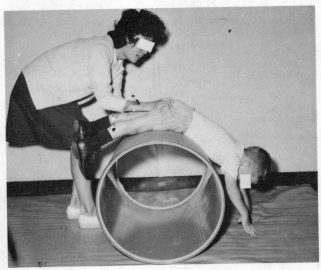

**A**   **B**

**FIG. 2-2.** Barrel (*A*) supporting boy as he is assisted in rolling over to touch floor (*B*). (From Denhoff, E., and Langdon, M., eds. Cerebral dysfunction: A treatment program for young children. *Clin Pediat 5*:332, 1966. (Reproduced with permission)

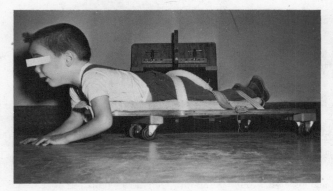

**FIG. 2-3.** Clinic-designed creeper that enables child to propel himself by his hands. (Courtesy of A. Slominski, Cerebral Palsy Clinic, Indiana University Medical Center)

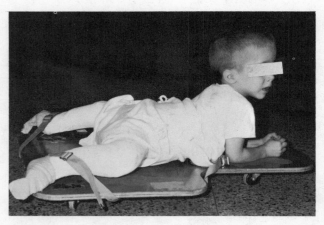

**FIG. 2-4.** Scoot-A-Bout, propelled by arm action, suitable for child in cast. (Courtesy of Central Wisconsin Colony, Madison, Wis.)

### Construction

1. Use 5-ply plywood (Fig. 2-5).
2. Overall measurements are 36 by 26 inches (Fig. 2-6).
3. Attach four 2-inch hard rubber casters (*C*).
4. Attach three adjustable straps across bottom of board, at the two lower corners, to hold the legs, and at the center where the board narrows for the chest, to hold the trunk in position.

### SCOOT-A-BOUT PC 4762

The Scoot-A-Bout (Fig. 2-7) is propelled by use of the arms. The leg pads are adjustable in height and in leg spread to accommodate leg length and cast contours. The crawler is constructed of chrome-plated steel with spherical casters and foam-cushioned body and leg pads; safety belts are attached. Overall length is 36 inches and minimal height from the floor is 6 inches. The body pad is 9 by 20½ inches; leg pads attached to body pad are 6¼ by 8¼ inches; the end leg pads are 6¼ by 10¼ inches.

### Source

J. A. Preston Corp.

### CRAWLER PC 4541

This crawler (Fig. 2-8) can be propelled by the arms or legs or both. It has an all-steel chassis, an adjustable canvas pad to support the chest and abdomen, and an adjustable and detachable armrest. The finish is bright red enamel.

### Source

J. A. Preston Corp.

### ADAPTIVE CREEPER

Made of tubular steel construction, this creeper adjusts to accommodate an average 2- to 8-year-old child. It may be propelled by the arms or legs or both, and will support a weight up to 250 pounds.

### Source

Adaptive Creepers

### HOSPITAL-MADE CRAWLER

A hospital-made crawler, constructed of welded pipe, has wide canvas straps that may be adjusted to support the child at three points (Fig. 2-9).

## STANDING AIDS

### STANDING SUPPORT

A child may be assisted to stand by supporting the legs with magazines that are tied around them by broad bands with bows (Fig. 2-10). Further support to prevent falling is supplied by using a diaper or dishtowel around the waist and chest, held by an adult.

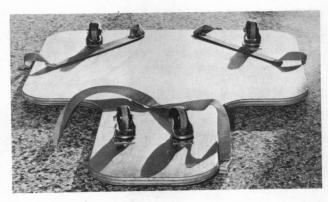

**FIG. 2-5.** Underside of Scoot-A-Bout, showing attachment of straps and casters. (Courtesy of Central Wisconsin Colony, Madison, Wis.)

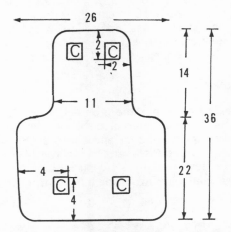

**FIG. 2-6.** Diagram for construction of Scoot-A-Bout and placement of casters, *C,* and straps. (Courtesy of Central Wisconsin Colony, Madison, Wis.)

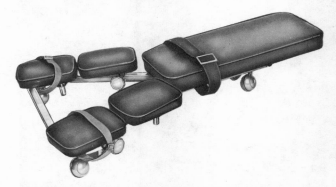

**FIG. 2-7.** Scoot-A-Bout PC 4762, to be propelled by use of arms. (Copyright 1965 by J. A. Preston Corporation)

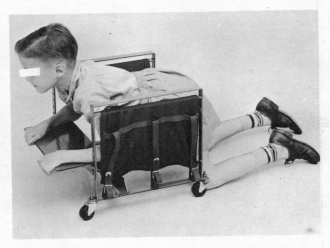

**FIG. 2-8.** Crawler PC 4541, to be propelled by use of arms or legs or both. (Copyright 1965 by J. A. Preston Corporation)

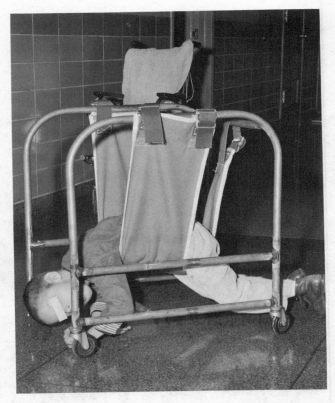

**FIG. 2-9.** Hospital-made crawler, supporting child who is using both arms and legs to move about. (Courtesy of R. Wiley, United Cerebral Palsy of Southwest Missouri)

## PRONE-STANDER

A useful device for both self-locomotion and assisted transport is the prone-stander (Fig. 2-11). The child may lie on the board and propel himself with his arms (Fig. 2-11*A*). In this position, the hands are well behind the front wheels of the board. With the detachable footboard in place (Fig. 2-11*B*) and the prone-stander partially upraised, an adult can transport the child. Since the child is held securely to the board by broad bands, the prone-stander can be placed in an upright position (Fig. 2-11*C*) for transport or standing.

### Precautions

1. If an adult is not holding the upright board while the child is standing on it, it must be secured to a wall or stable object by means of D rings.
2. When the patient uses the prone-stander in an upright position, he should be turned so that his back is against the board.

### Construction

The basic structure of the prone-stander (Fig. 2-12) consists of a rectangular piece of ¾-inch plywood padded with sponge rubber and covered with Naugahyde. A detachable footboard is secured to the main board with metal braces and wing nuts. It can be removed by unlatching two door hinges at the bottom.

**FIG. 2-10.** A diaper or dishtowel used about child's body, enabling her to stand. Her legs are supported by magazines tied in place. (From Denhoff, E., and Langdon, M., eds. Cerebral dysfunction: A treatment program for young children. *Clin. Pediat 5:*332, 1966. Reproduced with permission)

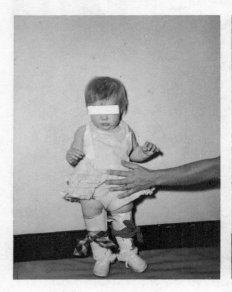
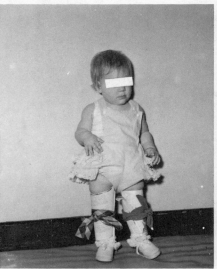
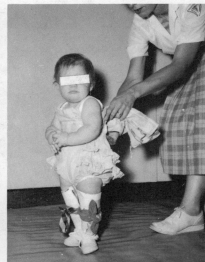

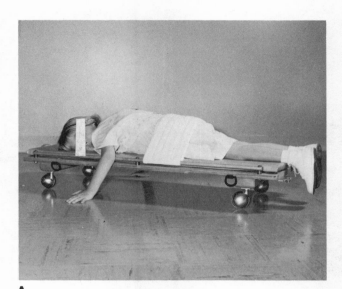

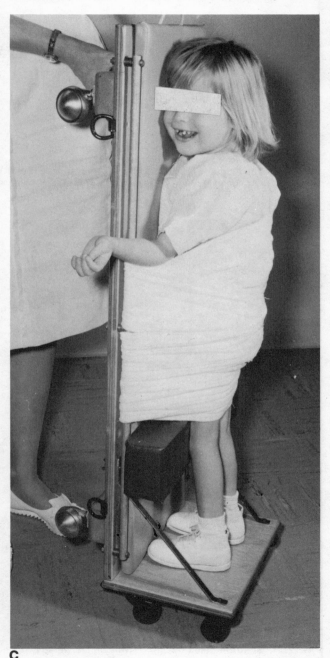

**FIG. 2-11.** Prone stander in position for locomotion by use of arms (*A*); with footrest down and prone-stander in partially upright position for assisted transportation (*B*); and in fully upright position (*C*). (Courtesy of Physical Therapy Department, Rancho Los Amigos Hospital, Downey, Calif. Reproduced with permission of *Physical Ther 47*:386, 1967)

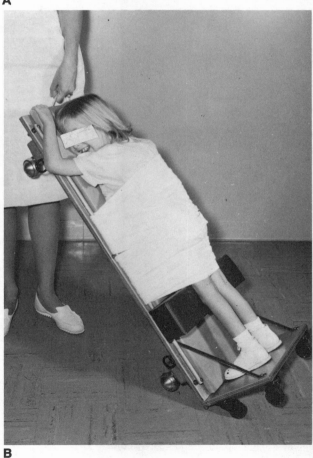

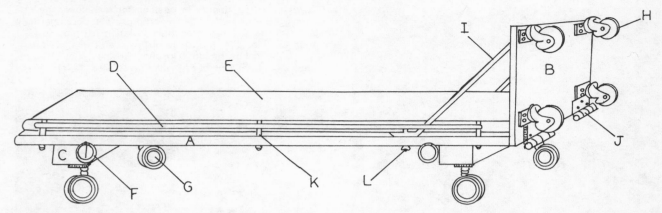

**FIG. 2-12.** Diagram for construction of prone-stander. Board, *A,* and detachable footboard, *B;* board braces and caster supports, *C;* pipe support, *D;* foam rubber pad, *E;* D rings, *F,* Shepherd casters, *G,* standard casters, *H,* braces for footboard, *I;* door hinges, *J,* 2-inch bolts, *K,* and smaller bolts with wing nuts, *L.* (Courtesy of Physical Therapy Department, Rancho Los Amigos Hospital, Downey, Calif. Reproduced with permission of *Physical Ther 47:*386, 1967)

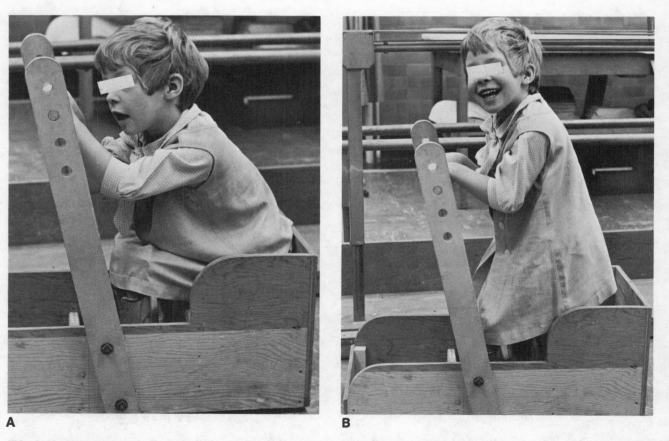

**FIG. 2-13.** Sit-down-stand-up chair with child seated (*A*) and pulling herself up to stand (*B*). (Courtesy of A. Slominski, Cerebral Palsy Clinic, Indiana University Medical Center)

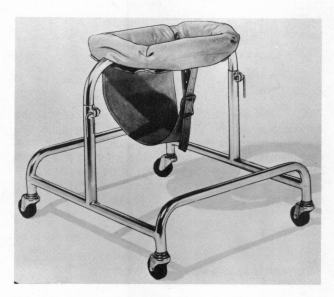

**FIG. 2-14.** Infant walker PC 1763S. (Copyright 1965 by J. A. Preston Corporation)

The main board and footboard are fitted with Shepherd casters or caster wheels on each corner.

Metal rods run the length of the board, and are used to secure ties or straps to hold the patient in the desired position. Two D rings on each side of the board near the top and bottom are used to secure it in the upright position. A handle of rope or leather at the top facilitates raising the device to the upright position. When the board is used for standing, a pad may be placed at the knees.

1. Board (*A*). Use ¾-inch plywood, 14 by 40 inches.
2. Footboard (*B*). Use ¾-inch plywood, 10 by 14 inches.
3. Board braces (*C*), two pieces. Use pine stock, 1½ by 2¾ by 13¾ inches. Attach to board (*A*) with six No. 8 1½-inch flathead screws.
4. Rods (*D*). Use two pieces of pipe, ½-inch outside diameter, 36 inches long.
5. Pad (*E*). Use foam rubber, 1 inch thick by 11½ by 40 inches. Cover with leatherette and glue to board (*A*).
6. D rings (*F*). Secure four rings to plywood by four flat iron pieces curled into a loop on one end. Pieces should be ⅛ inch by ¾ by 3½ inches.
7. Shepherd casters (*G*). Attach four casters to board braces (*C*) with wood screws.
8. Conventional casters (*H*). Attach four casters to footboard (*B*) with wood screws.
9. Braces (*I*). Use flat iron pieces, ⅛ inch by ½ inch by 14 inches, angled to 45 degrees on both ends.
10. Door hinges (*J*) with removable pins. Use 1½- by 3½-inch size.
11. Bolts (*K*). Use six 2-inch bolts with ½-inch spacers (or several washers) to attach pipe (*D*) to board *A*.
12. Bolts (*L*) with wing nuts. Use two 1¼-inch bolts to attach braces (*I*) to board (*A*).

### SIT-DOWN-STAND-UP CHAIR

This chair (Fig. 2-13) is useful for a child learning to pull himself up to a standing position and to stand still.

## WALKING LEARNING AIDS

Walkers are useful in selected situations as aids to ambulation and independence. The physician in charge of the child's developmental program should be consulted to determine whether a walker is indicated and, if so, how much support it should provide. Several types of walkers are available, with balance ring and optional seating, adjustable within a few sizes.

### Sources

G. E. Miller, Inc.
Orthopedic Services of Rhode Island
J. A. Preston Corp.
American Hospital Supply
Scully Walton (Rents as well as sells equipment).

### INFANT WALKER PC 1763S

Designed for children between the ages of 1½ years and 4 years, this walker (Fig. 2-14) is adjustable in height from 18 to 24 inches. A padded balance ring and an adjustable saddle seat hold the child in an upright position. The overall width is 19 inches; the length, 20 inches.

### Source

J. A. Preston Corp.

### CHILD WALKER PC 1762

Suitable for children 2 to 8 years of age, this chromium-plated walker (Fig. 2-15) has handrails adjust-

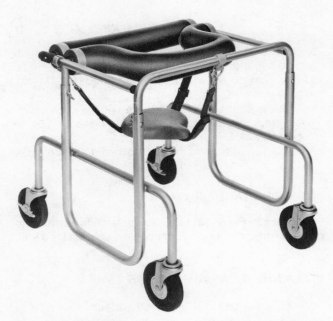

**FIG. 2-15.** Child walker PC 1762. (Copyright 1965 by J. A. Preston Corporation)

able in height from 23 to 31 inches. A padded body ring, with an inside diameter of 10 inches, opens in the rear for easy entrance and exit. The saddle seat is adjustable. There are four ball-bearing casters, two with step-on brakes.

### Source

J. A. Preston Corp.

### CHILDREN'S TRAINING WALKER PC 1759

A small-size walker (Fig. 2-16) has a rib belt attachment only. All four casters have step-on brakes.

### Source

J. A. Preston Corp.

### CHILDREN'S TRAINING WALKER PC 1760

This walker (Fig. 2-17) has a balance ring and saddle seat; all casters have step-on brakes. A similar model (PC 1761) comes with a rib belt attachment, balance ring, and saddle seat. A large-size training walker (PC 1759J) has a rib belt attachment only; the PC 1760J is the same with a balance ring and saddle seat only; and the PC 1761J is the same with all three attachments—rib belt, balance ring, and saddle seat.

### Source

J. A. Preston Corp.

### SLED CHAIR

A special back unit, consisting of runners, can be added to a regular chair (Fig. 2-18). The child can push the chair as he learns to walk. The back unit, which stops the chair from tipping, must have a length one and a half times the height of the chair to be effective. A center board discourages foot and leg adduction.

### Precaution

Pad the top bar of the chair back to prevent injury if the pusher should fall against the chair.

### STURDY PUSHER

This pusher (Fig. 2-19) has a low center of gravity that makes it sturdy. The handle is adjustable in height. While the child is being aided to walk, this unit provides nursery fun, too.

### PARALLEL BARS

For the handicapped child learning to walk on his own or with an aid, parallel bars are often useful for training and practice.

**FIG. 2-16.** Children's training walker PC 1759. (Copyright 1965 by J. A. Preston Corporation)

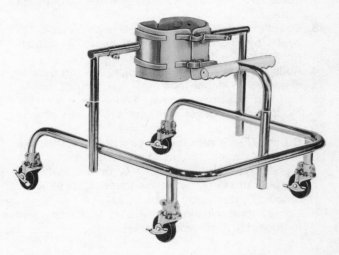

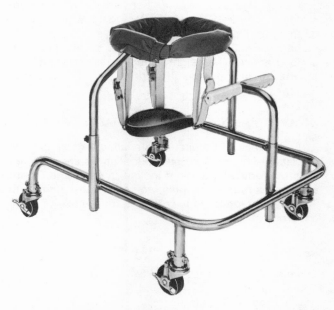

**FIG. 2-17.** Children's training walker PC 1760. (Copyright 1965 by J. A. Preston Corporation)

**FIG. 2-18.** Sled chair made from regular chair with back runners added. (Courtesy of University of California, Developmental Center, Los Angeles)

**FIG. 2-19.** Sturdy pusher, with adjustable handle. (Courtesy of A. Slominski, United Cerebral Palsy Clinic, Indiana University Medical Center)

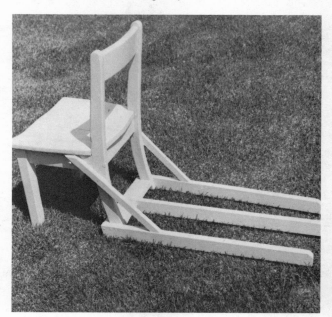

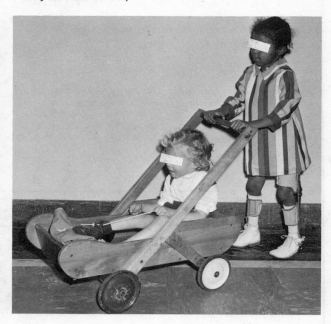

### Construction

Parallel bars may be constructed to suit the needs of a particular group of children or adults (Fig. 2-20).

1. Base. Use two pieces of hardwood, 1½ by 8 by 26 inches, with lengthwise edges (*A-B* and *C-D*) beveled to prevent the user from tripping at entrance and exit.
2. Uprights. Four pieces of iron pipe, 1¼ inches outside diameter and 20 inches long.
3. Flanges. Four iron flanges are needed for 1¼-inch pipe.
4. Reducers. Four, of iron, 1¼ inches reducing to 1 inch. Ream the 1-inch ends to slide into adjustable uprights.
5. Adjustable uprights. Four pieces of iron pipe, 1 inch outside diameter, and 20 inches long. The length of these uprights may be adjusted to the patient's height. A lower bar may be added for smaller children using the same equipment.
6. Bars. Four pieces of iron pipe, 1 inch outside diameter and 84 inches long.
7. Elbows. Four, of iron, for 1-inch pipe.
8. Thumb screws. Four, of steel, ⅜ inch in diameter, with cupped point. If the joint between the flanges and the uprights is not too tight, the bars may be folded together when not in use.

### Precautions

1. Base should be anchored to the floor for heavy people.
2. A rubber floor mat is recommended between uprights for the length of the walk.

**FIG. 2-20.** Diagram for construction of parallel bars that are adjustable in height. (*1*) Base with edges *A-B* and *C-D* beveled. (*2*) Upright. (*3*) Flange. (*4*) Reducer. (*5*) Adjustable upright section. (*6*) Bars. (*7*) Elbow. (*8*) Thumb screw. (Courtesy of C. Maciulewicz, United Cerebral Palsy Association, Erie, Pa.)

### PARALLEL BARS WITH FEET SEPARATOR

Another type of parallel bars that may be constructed (Fig. 2-21) has a center board which serves to separate the feet. The design of this 7-foot-long set of bars is a little simpler than that of the bars described above. The height should be made adjustable to the height of the handgrips of the patient's crutches.

### COMMERCIALLY AVAILABLE PARALLEL BARS

Some types of parallel bars available commercially are stationary and floor-mounted. Others are mounted on a platform with a slight incline at each end. There are two pairs of hand rails, adjustable in height, and 10 to 12 feet long; the lower set is for the use of small children.

### Sources

Hausmann Industries, Inc.
G. E. Miller, Inc.
J. A. Preston Corp.

## WALKING AIDS

### RECIPROCAL WALKER

The reciprocal walker (Fig. 2-22) comes in three sizes and can be weighted with lead to provide greater support for the athetoid.

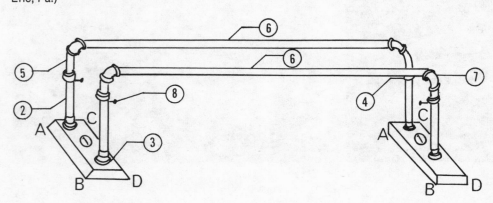

## Source

Anita Slominski, OTR, Coordinator

## WALKER WITH BRAKES

This walker (Fig. 2-23) has hand brakes that can be used by the patient or the therapist. The brakes can be attached to one bar if only one hand is functional. A seat can be added, and the walker can be weighted if necessary.

## Source

Anita Slominski, OTR, Coordinator

## QUAD CANE

The quad cane (Fig. 2-24) is lightweight and yet provides stability for the unsteady walker.

## Source

Anita Slominski, OTR, Coordinator

## CRUTCHES

Crutches and canes must be selected and fitted by the medical team. There is a considerable variety from which to choose:
1. Wood or aluminum ones
2. Adjustable aluminum or wood ones
3. Tripod cane, sometimes called a "crab cane," or cane glider
4. Canadian crutches
5. Lofstrand crutches
6. Walker type crutches

## Sources

Everest & Jennings, Inc.
Lumex, Inc.
G. E. Miller, Inc.
Orthopedic Equipment Co.
J. A. Preston Corp.
American Hospital Supply

## CRUTCH AIDS

A few crutch aids (Fig. 2-25) have been found particularly useful: Deluxe Crutch Tip PC 7336S-L-M; Safe-T-Fex crutch tip PC 7336; and ice grippers PC 7340, which may be used in all weather.

## Source

J. A. Preston Corp.

## MATHENY SCHOOL CRUTCH CONTROL

A crutch control suitable for either children or adults (Fig. 2-26) is the Matheny School Crutch Control. It may be used with wood or aluminum crutches of either standard or Canadian type, and is easily adjusted and transferred from one set of crutches to another. The crutch control eliminates the crossing of the crutches and controls the arm swing and ultimate placement of each crutch. The standard model has

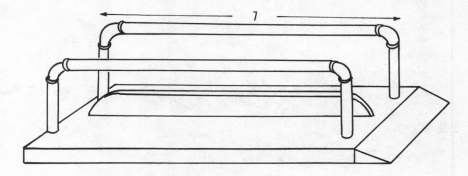

**FIG. 2-21.** Diagram for construction of parallel bars that are not adjustable in height and have a feet divider. (Courtesy of Cerebral Palsy Unit, New York State Rehabilitation Hospital, West Haverstraw, N.Y.)

7

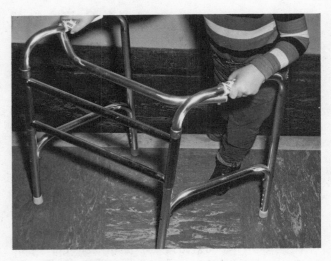

**FIG. 2-22.** Reciprocal walker, adaptable for athetoids. (Courtesy of A. Slominski, Cerebral Palsy Clinic, Indiana University Medical Center)

**FIG. 2-23.** Walker with brakes. Therapist has her hand on the brakes. (Courtesy of A. Slominski, Cerebral Palsy Clinic, Indiana University Medical Center)

**FIG. 2-24.** Quad canes to aid unsteady walker. (Courtesy of A. Slominski, Cerebral Palsy Clinic, Indiana University Medical Center)

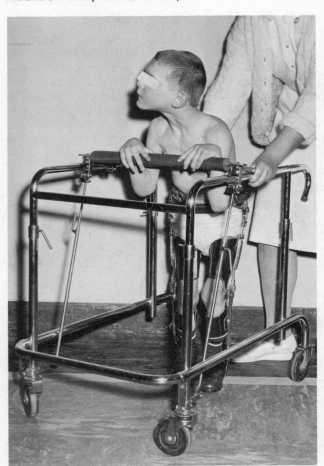

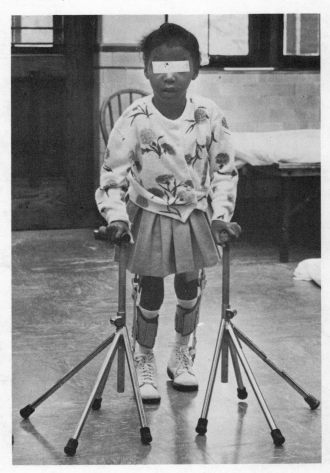

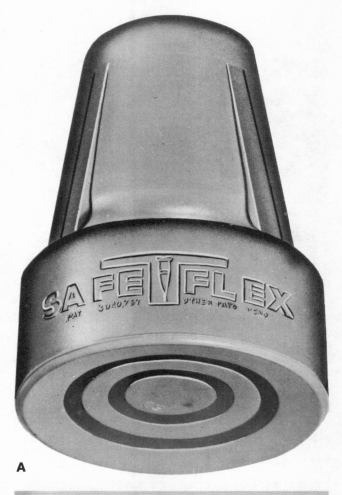

**A**

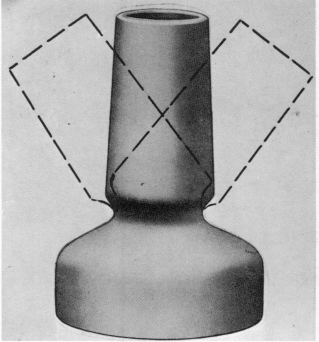

**B**

FIG. 2-25. Crutch aids. (*A*) Deluxe crutch tip PC 7336S-L-M. (*B*) Safe-T-Flex crutch tip PC 7336. (*C*) Ice grippers PC 7340, shown in position for use on ice and snow at left and in position for normal use at right. (Copyright 1965 by J. A. Preston Corporation)

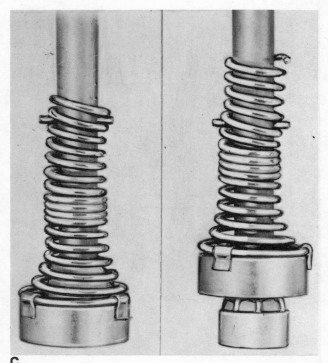

**C**

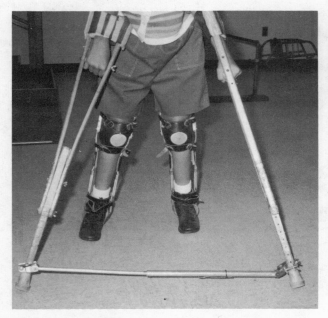

**FIG. 2-26.** Matheny School Crutch Control, easily adjustable and transferable from one set of crutches to another. (Courtesy of the Matheny School, Peapack, N.J.)

**FIG. 2-27.** Diagram for crutch holder for desk, with a 7-inch bracket at top for wider part of crutches and a 4-inch bracket for the lower part. (Courtesy of the New York University Medical Center, Institute of Rehabilitation Medicine, New York, N.Y.)

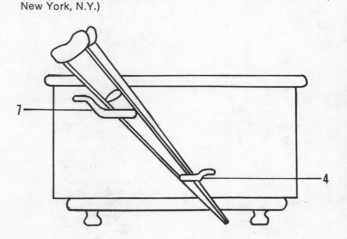

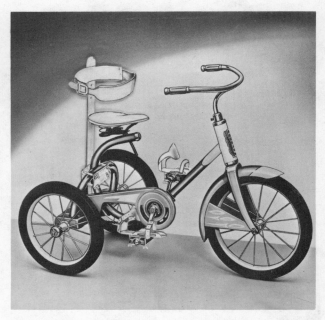

**FIG. 2-28.** Tricycle with body support bolted to frame, and foot support on pedals. (Copyright 1965 by J. A. Preston Corporation)

**FIG. 2-29.** Built-up chair for back support. Seat belt holds child in place. (Courtesy of G. Fullan, Spastic Aid of Alabama, Inc., Birmingham)

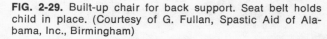

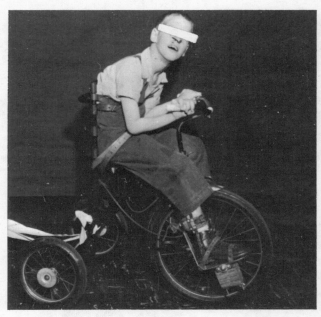

a minimum spread of 22½ inches and a maximum spread of 37 inches. There are also special sizes, within limits, on request.

## Sources

D. C. Denison Orthopaedic Appliance Corp.
J. A. Preston Corp.

## CRUTCH HOLDER FOR DESK

A crutch holder (Fig. 2-27) suitable for a desk, and possibly adaptable for other places, is a highly useful device to keep the desk worker's crutches within convenient reach but where they will not be a hazard to others. The crutch holder is not available commercially, but was designed by and for Pan American Airways, Long Island City, N.Y.

## Construction

1. Two aluminum brackets are needed, one 7 inches long and the other 4 inches.
2. Attach the longer bracket to one side of the desk near the top, to accommodate the widest part of the crutches.
3. Attach the shorter bracket to the desk near the bottom of the opposite edge of the desk side. It should be a sufficient distance from the top bracket to permit the crutches to rest at a convenient angle.

# TRICYCLES

A tricycle, sturdily built and incorporating special safety features, can provide excellent exercise and training for the handicapped child while he enjoys great fun wheeling it about.

## Sources

Adultrike Manufacturing Co. (Division of Custom Cycle)
J. J. Block (built-up chain velocipede and built-up chain drive tricycle)
Gobby Manufacturing, Inc.
The Huffman Manufacturing Co.
J. A. Preston Corp. (tricycle with body support)
Schwinn Bicycle Co.

## Precautions

1. Be sure that tricycle is sturdy, with a wide base to prevent tipping.
2. Use a chair guard and adjustable seat, for safety and posture.
3. Use body support and foot attachment (Fig. 2-28). If body support is needed, see that it does not push the child off the seat. Check to see that when it is in place, the child's buttocks rest squarely on the bike seat at its widest part, not on the narrow front section.
4. Use padding in the middle of the handle bars for the unsteady child.

## BUILT-UP CHAIR BACK FOR SEAT

Some tricycles have a built-up chair back for greater security (Fig. 2-29). With adapted foot pedals, and a padded midsection on the handlebar, the non-ambulatory child is able to get about indoors and outside. In Figure 2-29 the overall positioning of the pedaler leaves something to be desired, but his new capacity to function is developmentally sound.

## PEDAL HOLDER

Rubber bands cut from automobile tire inner tube can be used to hold a child's feet onto tricycle pedals (Fig. 2-30). In the illustration, the weight of the shoe has caused it to drop, turning the pedal over. In use, however, the child's foot remains on top of the pedal.

# WALKING CHAIR

This prototype of a new "walking chair" (Fig. 2-31) was designed to give more mobility to the disabled child. It is being evaluated at the Rehabilitation Center of the University of California at Los Angeles. The original concept came from a Moonwalker proposed by Space General Corporation for initial exploration of the moon, as part of the Centaur-Surveyor program.

It is included in this manual as an illustration of the way in which rehabilitation planning looks toward all sources for the ideas for aids.

# PROTECTIVE HELMETS

The use of a protective helmet can help to spare the child from further injury when he falls.

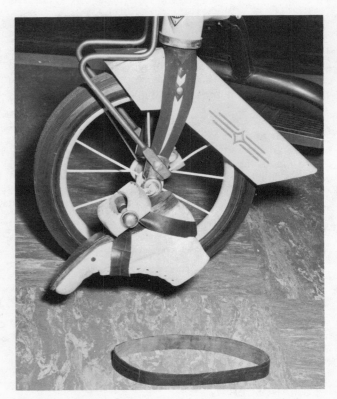

## LEATHER HELMETS

Most commercial helmets (Figs. 2-32 and 2-33) are made in sizes 18 through 25, with special sizes made to order. Cycling helmets have also proved useful. For a child who is inclined to fall and bruise his chin, a football chin guard may be attached to the helmet, using hammer-on snaps.

### Sources

Bacharach-Rasin
J. A. Preston Corp.
Stall & Dean Manufacturing Co.

## CLOTH HELMETS

A commercially produced helmet is available in two styles, made of plain or striped denim, at modest prices.

### Source

Vocational Guidance and Rehabilitation Services

### Construction

A protective headgear can be made at home from plastic sponge (Fig. 2-34). The pattern is simple and easily followed (Fig. 2-35).

**FIG. 2-30.** Pedal holders attached to shoe by bands cut from auto inner tube. (From Bensberg, G. J., ed. *Teaching the Mentally Retarded: A Handbook for Ward Personnel.* Atlanta, Ga., Southern Regional Education Board, 1966. Reproduced with permission)

**FIG. 2-31.** Walking chair, designed on lines of a Moonwalker. (Courtesy of Space-General Corporation, El Monte, Calif.)

**FIG. 2-32.** Solid-crown helmet, offering maximum protection to front and back of head. (Courtesy of Stall & Dean, Brockton, Mass.)

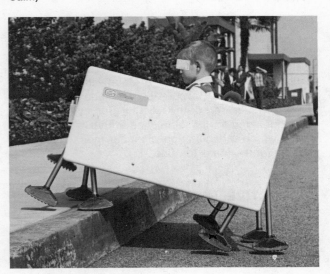

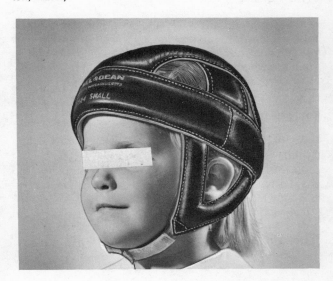

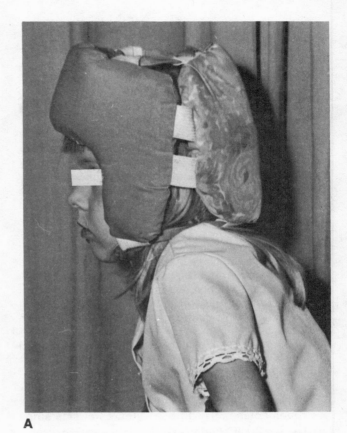

A

**FIG. 2-33.** Soft-crown helmet, offering maximum protection to front, back, and top of head. (Courtesy of Stall & Dean, Brockton, Mass.)

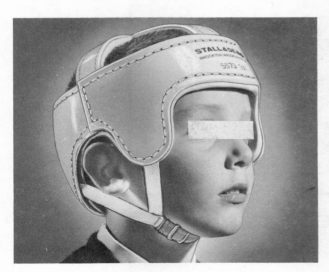

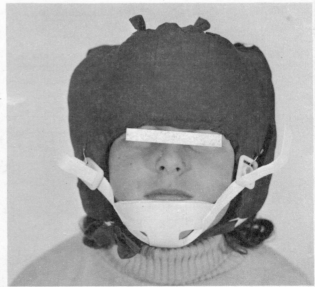

B

**FIG. 2-34.** (*A*) Helmet made of plastic sponge, covered with cotton. (*B*) Plastic chin protector attached to helmet. (Courtesy of A. Slominski, Cerebral Palsy Clinic, Indiana University Medical Center. Reproduced with permission)

1. Allow ½-inch seam allowance on all pieces, including elastic.
2. Eight strips of 1¼-inch webbed elastic cut 2 inches long are needed for loops (L).
3. Four strips of 1¼-inch webbed elastic cut 1 inch long are needed for side strips (S).
4. Use calico or denim, or other moderately heavy cotton. Cut two pieces for the front (F) and two for the back (B).
5. Place right sides of the two front pieces (F) together and pin ends of the 2-inch elastic to form loops (L) between the two surfaces. Pin one end of 1-inch side elastic (S) between the two surfaces.
6. Cut sponge padding, one piece to pattern of front piece (F) to fit inside dotted seam allowance.
7. Sew around front (F) pieces, leaving area between notches (N-N) open so that sponge can be added. Turn and press. After sponge padding has been added, turn in remaining seam allowance and top stitch between notches.
8. Place right sides of back pieces (B) together and pin ends of 2-inch elastic to form loops (L), just as with front, but wait until sponge has been inserted to sew in the two back neck loops.
9. Sew around back pieces (B), leaving area between notches (N-N) open and area of side strips (S) open. Turn and press.
10. Insert side strips of front (F) into areas for back

side strips, turn in seam allowance and top stitch back (B) over side strips. Insert sponge padding, turn in seam allowance and pin in neck loops. Top stitch.
11. Cut two straps, one for the top (TS) and one for the neck (NS). Fold each lengthwise, right sides together. Stitch seam and turn and press. Snip neck strap (NS) in half and recombine it by means of a snap. Then turn in seam allowances on the ends of the two straps and top stitch.
12. The shorter strap (TS) is run through the four upper loops of the helmet and tied in a bow. The chin strap (NS) is run through the loops at the neck and chin and tied under the chin.

### Precaution

The snap opening at the center back of the chin strap is essential. An adult can unsnap this easily if child ever gets caught or his position makes the bow at the throat too tight.

## MATS

Fitted equipment is fine, but there is also a time and place for being relaxed and unsupported, for free movement and for play. For these purposes, mats are perfect.

**FIG. 2-35.** Diagram for making helmet of plastic sponge. Front, *F*, and back, *B*, showing points for loops, *L*, and side strips, *S*. Notches, *N*; top strap, *TS*; neck strap, *NS*. Dotted line indicates ½-inch seam allowance for cloth and outside dimensions for cutting sponge rubber pad. (Courtesy of A. Slominski, Cerebral Palsy Clinic, Indiana University Medical Center)

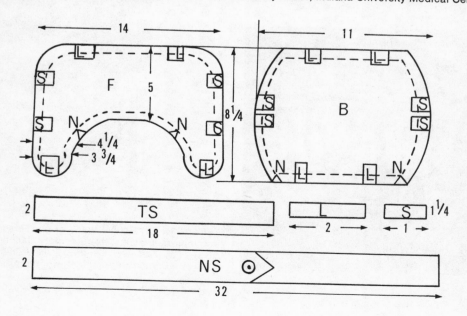

**Sources**

G. E. Miller, Inc.
Nissen Corp. (Exercise Pads)
J. A. Preston Corp.

# REFERENCES

Bensberg, G. J., ed. *Teaching the Mentally Retarded: A Handbook for Ward Personnel.* Atlanta, Southern Regional Education Board, 1966.

Denhoff, E., Langdon, M., eds. "Cerebral dysfunction: A treatment program for young children," Clin Pediat 5: 332, 1966.

# 3
# Wheelchairs and Adaptations

Every wheelchair buyer should seek competent medical advice. Good value does not necessarily mean low cost. Good value means, rather, that the chair *fits* the person and is useful.

**General Considerations**

In selecting a wheelchair, the buyer should weigh whether the chair will:
1. Ease the patient's disability
2. Promote his ability to function as adequately as possible
3. Be durable for inside and/or outside activities
4. Be strong and durable for persons with uncontrolled motion
5. Be lightweight and folding, for easy transport
6. Be adapted with accessories that, preferably, can be easily made or can be purchased and replaced
7. Have brakes and seat belts

Since each wheelchair recommendation is an individual one (there is no average case of cerebral palsy), there will be many factors to consider (Fig. 3-1). Before making a final decision, check the following points:
1. The patient's accurate measurements
2. Accurate measurements of the chair

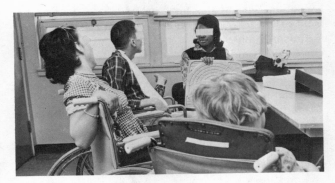

**FIG. 3-1.** Each Wheelchair recommendation is an individual one. (Courtesy of United Cerebral Palsy of Denver)

3. Position of the user's feet on the footrests, so that they rest securely
4. Adaptations that may be necessary to alleviate extensor thrust, tonic neck reflex, poor head control, poor trunk control when sitting
5. Adaptations that may be needed for transfer of the patient from the wheelchair to bed, toilet, etc.
6. Suitability of the chair for the setup of the home or wherever the user will spend the most time or have the greatest need for the chair
7. Ease of cleaning and maintenance
8. Availability of repair services

In the References section of this chapter are listed the names and addresses of a number of manufacturers and distributors of wheelchairs. Graduated sizes of wheelchairs are available—those for the tiny tot, junior age, the "growing" chair, adult size, and heavy duty. They should be ordered by *size* and not by age. Some tips on proper measuring may be found in the measurement blank supplied by the J. A. Preston Corp. or the form supplied by Everest & Jennings, Inc.

In weighing the purchase of a wheelchair or other equipment, particularly for the growing child, it would be well to consider rental or to investigate possible sources of loan equipment, providing that all needs can be well met by the equipment available. United Cerebral Palsy of Greater Kansas is one organization maintaining an equipment pool. In their annual report for 1967 they state:

"Equipment Pool programming began years ago with the donations from parents of usable but outgrown equipment. Now more than 176 items with an estimated value of $8,500 are loaned free of charge to children in the Greater Kansas area. We are most appreciative of the efforts by the Kansas City Housewares Club whose annual 'Sample Sale' proceeds enable this agency to replenish our equipment pool stock."

Do not order a wheelchair until all uses and all possible adaptations that may be needed are considered.

## ANSWERS TO COMMON QUESTIONS

### HOW YOUNG A CHILD CAN GO INTO A WHEELCHAIR?

This cannot be answered by generalities. Members of the child's medical team can advise you. Children as young as 3 years have been fitted for wheelchairs when the prognosis for walking seemed poor. They are useful when a child is especially large or heavy, when the parent is unable to lift or carry the child, and for convenience in feeding the child.

### HOW CAN A WHEELCHAIR BE MADE ECONOMICALLY FEASIBLE FOR A SMALL CHILD OR A RAPIDLY GROWING CHILD?

One suggestion is to use upholstery that will narrow the width of the chair yet allow it to expand with the child, as needed. Wooden inserts made to fit can also provide firm adjustments. In making such adaptations, it is essential to have the advice and guidance of a fitting expert—nurse or therapist.

### WHAT ABOUT PUSH CHAIRS THAT ARE NOT WHEELCHAIRS?

There is nothing like a well-fitted wheelchair for optimum function. However, some of the inexpensive push chairs do come in handy for *transporting* the nonambulatory child whose prognosis for walking may be good but who needs to be taken from one location to another by an adult. Some have been found useful at beaches, where an expensive chair might be damaged.

Some athetoid children experience distress in those chairs which must be tilted back in order to be moved, for it disturbs their already precarious balance. Therefore, all use of temporary pushers should depend

---

Many ideas in this chapter have been contributed by therapists collaborating in teams around the country. See Legends of figures for specific credits.

upon the effects upon the patient. Temporary push chairs will never be a stubstitute for a wheelchair and are unsatisfactory for the child who must spend long periods in a wheelchair since the nature of the push chair's construction does not lend itself well to adapting it to fit individual needs. Nor do the chairs last long enough to justify the time or money to make adaptations.

## DOES IT MATTER WHERE THE BRAKES ARE PUT?

The position of brakes and their length depends on the hand use and arm strength of the user.

## WHAT SIZE SHOULD CASTERS BE?

Casters with an 8-inch diameter usually allow greater maneuverability and stability on less-than-smooth surfaces.

## WHY DO SOME CHAIRS HAVE DIFFERENT ARMS AND ARMRESTS?

In the past, detachable armrests were ordered less frequently for individuals with cerebral palsy since it takes good eye-hand coordination to manage them. If a person does not need the leverage and support of regular armrests and if he spends the bulk of his time at desks, tables, or work areas, it may be useful to have desk arms on his wheelchair—arms with a lower front portion that allow the chair to be moved close to the desk or table. However, detachable armrests may help parents to transfer the patient sideways out of the chair. Lately, Everest and Jennings has begun carrying detachable armrests which adjust in height. This is invaluable for use on a growing wheelchair as proper arm/tray height is always insured. It should be considered when ordering all types of wheelchairs now.

### Source

Everest and Jennings, Inc. Standard arm 25 ADA, Desk arm 26 ADA (no extra charge for these as basic armrest deducted).

## WHAT ADAPTATIONS HELP POSTURE AND FUNCTION?

No adaptation guarantees help; each must be fitted to the individual and tried with the idea of trying something else if the first effort does not succeed. Most of the following suggestions were developed by P. Holser-Buehler, and A. Wolfe, UCPA Consultants of Los Angeles and Don Guetts of Abbey Rents.

1. Heel straps, wider or deeper footrests, or heel or toe loops may help the patient to rest his feet more securely on the footrests. Plastic tubing encircling the back of the footrest, into which the feet are inserted, is helpful, does the same job as toe and heel loops, and can be quickly and inexpensively replaced.
2. Contoured back supports, wedge cushions, or plywood inserts sometimes prove helpful in counteracting extension patterns found in some severely handicapped children (see Figures 3-6 and 3-8).
3. Occasionally cushions or foam rubber on boards cut out at pressure areas may be recommended by the therapist (see Figure 3-21).
4. A wheelchair tray gives additional support to arms and so aids physical function and relaxation (Fig. 3-2).*

**FIG. 3-2.** Adjusto Tray attached to wheelchair, holding child securely in place. (Courtesy of P. Holser Buehler, Los Angeles, Calif.)

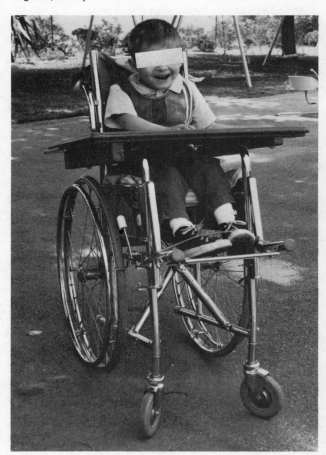

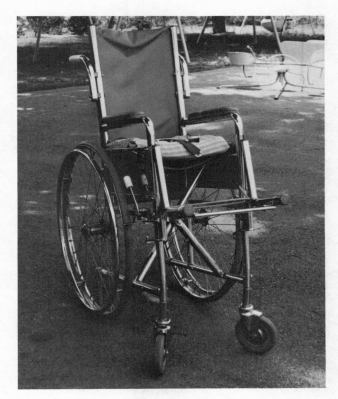

**FIG. 3-3.** Modified Wheelchair-Growing chair. Courtesy of P. Holser Buehler, Los Angeles, Calif.)

5. A padded wooden backrest gives better support than the leather upholstery of a wheelchair. Furthermore, it places the patient in a more functional position and thus aids in relaxation and arm use.
6. Risers on the casters of the wheelchair may also be useful, to tilt the chair back for the child whose head and body tends to fall forward in the chair.
7. Other useful adaptations, such as head wings, knee blocks, and side supports are described later in this chapter and in Chapter 1 in the section on chairs.

## WHEELCHAIR MODIFICATIONS FOR YOUNG CHILDREN

### WHEELCHAIR-GROWING CHAIR AND POSTURE-90 JUNIOR WHEELCHAIR

For children 6 to 16 years of age, the Growing Chair can be narrowed to 12 inches in width by up-

* See Holser-Buehler, P. Wheelchair utility tray. *Amer J Occup Ther* 24:49–50, 1970.

holstery to fit a child as young as 3 years, becoming a Tiny Tot wheelchair in size. When the upholstery is narrowed to 12 inches on a growing chair, the back can be made any height, especially if the child needs head support. The push handles must be screwed or welded to uprights if head support is needed (Fig. 3-3). One should also consider a Posture-90 wheelchair for this type of child. This chair has an excellent head wings/rest.

### Source

Everest & Jennings, Inc.

### FOOTREST WITH TOE BLOCK

This solid footrest (see Figure 3-7) has proved more practical than the type which is standard on the Growing Chair. The child's feet do not slip through, nor does the footrest swivel out of place.

### TUBING FOR FOOTSTRAPS

Tubing of the sort used for intravenous administration of fluids can be used for handy footstraps. The tubing is wrapped around the back supports of the footrest to form loops. The feet are inserted to prevent their sliding backward or forward.

### SNAPS-STRAPS-RINGS

A narrow (½-inch) seat belt may be advisable so that undue pressure is not placed on the child's abdomen or chest, as with the standard 2-inch-wide auto seat belt and buckle so commonly used on wheelchairs. This belt has a swivel snap hook closure that assures positive safety as it cannot be accidentally opened by the child. However, the belt should be positioned on the chair, not on the child.

### Source

Everest & Jennings, Inc.

### CASTER EXTENSION J111T

Caster extensions may be added to the front casters to tilt the chair back. They are useful for a child whose head or trunk tends to fall forward or for a child who needs a reclining position for relaxation. Extensions can be up to 5 inches in length, but generally 2 to 3 inches are sufficient.

**Source**

Everest & Jennings, Inc.

## WEBBING BELT

As an alternative, a webbing belt, Scout or army, may be looped under the wheelchair seat. It should be brought up on both sides between the seat and the side of the wheelchair, near the back edge of the chair. It is then hooked so that webbing goes over the upper thighs at the junction with the pelvis. This webbing may be screwed to the most terminal screw of the seat for correct placement on child.

## WEDGE-SHAPED CUSHION FOR JACKKNIFE POSITION

This cushion, which can be easily made, is placed on the chair so that the widest part fits the front edge of the chair seat. It raises the knees slightly higher than the hips and is effective as an aid to relaxation, especially for children with involuntary motion or for those who tend to go into an extensor thrust. It will not cut off circulation.

### Construction

1. Cut a wedge of foam rubber to fit the front of the chair. Experimentation is needed to determine the height of the wedge, but for the 2- or 3-year-old child, a wedge height of 2 inches is usually required.
2. Cover the wedge with washable material.

## UTILITY TRAY WITH ELASTIC CORD FASTENERS

This tray (Fig. 3-4) easily attaches by means of elastic cords and nonslip surfaces which hold it firmly to the wheelchair armrests. The cut-out tray curve, which nearly encircles the user, comes in three sizes, 9, 11, and 13 inches.

The tray was developed by a team of occupational therapists (P. Holser-Buehler, L. Barber, S. Brodish and E. Warner) and a design engineer and has held up clinically when used by very involved patients for extended periods.

Special features include durable ABS plastic with a raised edge; adequate relaxation space for elbows on extenders; narrowing at extenders, to allow the user to reach the wheels of the chair easily; elastic loops that can be pulled under the wheelchair arms;

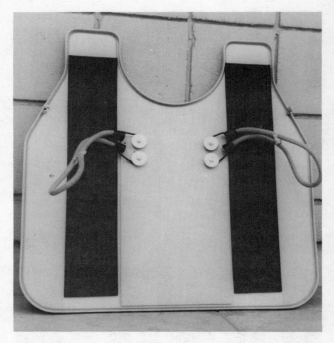

**FIG. 3-4.** Utility Tray, underside, showing the nonslip surfaces that protect armrests while adhering firmly, and the elastic loops that pass under chair arms and fasten tray at each side. (Courtesy of B&L Engineering, Downey, Calif.)

and a metal clip on each loop that hooks onto a clip underneath the tray at each side. A more recent model has additional strapping at extenders to prevent tray from flipping up at back and thus can be used on desk arms and new Everest and Jennings adjustable/detachable armrests.

**Source**

B & L Engineering
Distributed in major cities by Abbey Rents

## BOLT-ON HEADREST WITH HEADWINGS (4045 ADULT; 4045X JUNIOR)

These headwings can be bolted to solid insert back at desired height. The disadvantage is that they do not fit flush to the head.

**Source**

Everest & Jennings, Inc. (catalog contains picture of headwings).

## DETACHABLE HEADWINGS (J 415 TINY TOT)

The headwings are the same width as the chair. However, they do not fit flush to the head. They can be removed.

### Source

Everest & Jennings, Inc.

## SPECIAL SELF-CENTERING HEADREST 4045XAN

This is the same headrest as the one on the Posture-90 wheelchair (width of chair must be specified). The headrest can be adjusted in height and fits closely to the head. If the patient's head turns in one direction, that side can be padded to bring the head to the midline.

### Source

Everest & Jennings, Inc. (see catalog under Posture-90 for 4045 XAN headrest).

## SOLID INSERT BACKREST

Backrests should be considered an essential piece of equipment on wheelchairs for the patient with cerebral palsy since they place the patient in a more functional position and thus enhance relaxation and arm use. During the growing years, a child needs firm support for the back.

Solid insert back J4040, which is padded, is excellent when the child has no back problem. It fits all sizes of wheelchairs. Straps, which fasten to the push handles, hold the backrest in place.

### Source

Everest & Jennings, Inc.

**FIG. 3-5.** Outline of "T" backrest. T shape allows armrests to hold backrest in place without need for straps. (Courtesy of P. Holser Buehler, Los Angeles, Calif.)

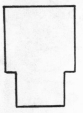

## POSTURE PANEL

A posture panel is good to correct improper posture of wheelchair patients, especially those who tend to slump forward.

### Source

J. A. Preston Corp. (see models PC 7077A, B, C, D in catalog for complete description)

## "T" BACKREST

This backrest is simple to make and is inexpensive (Fig. 3-5). It needs no straps to hold it in place, and it will not slide through the chair.

### Construction

1. Use ⅜-inch plywood. The height is the distance from the seat to the top of the upholstery on the back of the chair. It may be higher or lower, depending on the child's needs (many do best if the backrest comes only as high as their shoulders).
2. The width of the upper part of the backrest is measured from outside to outside of the back uprights.
3. The width of the lower part is 1 inch narrower on each side. The location of the 1-inch cut is determined by the distance from the seat to the *top* of the armrests.
4. Pad with 1-inch foam rubber, and cover with leatherette or washable material tacked in place for easy removal.

### Precautions

Take into consideration that the backrest will move the child forward in the chair since it rests in front of the back uprights. This alteration in position may cause the chair to fit improperly, and a tray may not fit either.

## INVERTED WHEELCHAIR BACK

A simple alteration in the back of a wheelchair that is upholstered may prove useful, giving support to the back of a child who cannot tolerate a regular backrest. However, it has some disadvantages: The upholstery wears out sooner, without board tending to deepen more than usual at the top of the chair; and inversion of the upholstery reduces the stability of the chair, which can be especially bad for the chair of a child with involuntary motion.

### Construction

1. Turn the upholstery on the back of the wheelchair upside down and screw back in place.
2. Open the upholstery at the edge, and insert a board ⅜ inch thick. The width of the board should be 1 inch less than the inside measurements of the back uprights.
3. Tack the upholstery shut and replace in back of the chair, still in an upside-down position.

## WHEELCHAIR MODIFICATIONS FOR THE SEVERELY DISABLED

In planning adaptive equipment for wheelchairs, many factors must be carefully considered to prevent harm or discomfort to the patient and to avoid costly errors. The following pointers are based upon information from the Cerebral Palsy Clinic of Indiana University Medical Center and the Warren G. Murray Children's Center, Centralia, Ill.

Team effort is required: All plans should be made and carried out in consultation with physicians, nurses, therapists, the family, and the carpenter. The patient's physical characteristics must be taken into account: head balance, trunk balance, degree of athetosis and extensor thrust, scissoring of legs (adduction), and scoliosis or other deformities affecting posture.

### MEASUREMENTS

1. Place the patient in a sitting position on a straight chair with a flat, firm seat.
2. Measure the patient with a yardstick, not a cloth tape. Follow the instructions given in Chapter 1 on Measurements for Special Equipment.

### POSTURE POINTERS

1. If it can be tolerated, the patient's back should be at a 90-degree angle.
2. A reclining back may be necessary for a weak child with poor trunk and head balance.
3. Side supports or head supports can be used (see Figures 3-6 and 3-8). The head support fits just above the shoulders and below the occipital area of the head. If the head support is too high, it may aggravate extensor thrust.

4. A vest can sometimes be used for trunk support. See Chapter 1, Vest for Trunk Support for directions to make a vest.
5. Padding should be eliminated as much as possible but, when necessary, is used for the following: (A) To prevent pressure areas. An athetoid may need padding for his arms and elbows, and in some instances of severe disability, he may need slots for wrist cuffs to stabilize his arms. (B) To prevent pressure on protruding bones. An opening may be cut in the seat or back, with padding as needed.
6. A rolled ventilated seat (patent pending) is contoured for comfort, and the body weight should be distributed along most of the thigh. An elevation of ¼ to 2 inches at the knees aids in control of scissoring or adduction.
7. A seat belt will help to ensure good posture. It should cross just in front of the bend in the hips when the patient is in a sitting position, to avoid undue constriction of the belt across the abdomen or chest. See the general instructions for seatbelts in Chapter 1 and under Wheelchair Safety Belts and Supports later in this chapter.

**FIG. 3-6.** Clinic-designed removable inserts: solid seat with padded wing supports, padded neck support, and padded backboard above neck support; rolled ventilated seat insert (patent pending) for hip flexion to inhibit hyperextension on the back; adjustable footrest with shoe holders; and safety belt of wide webbing. (Courtesy of A. Slominski, Cerebral Palsy Clinic, Indiana University Medical Center)

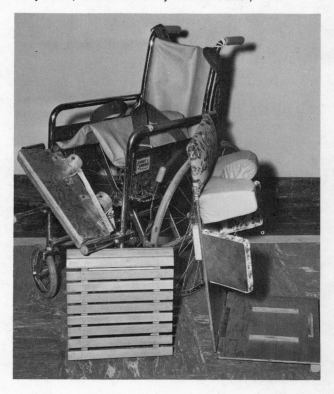

## AIDS IN CONTROLLING EXTENSOR THRUST

1. Pitch the back forward about 10 degrees (adjust at an 80-degree angle instead of the usual 90-degree angle).
2. Slant the seat to elevate the knees ½ to 2 inches.
3. Use a solid footrest and elevate the toes slightly, up to a maximum of 2 inches (see Fig. 3-7).
4. Eliminate pressure on the soles of the feet at the matatarsal-phalangeal joint.

## AIDS IN STABILIZING LIMBS

1. Use arm restraint straps.
2. Try stabilizing one arm. It may improve coordination of the other hand and arm.
3. Use heel and foot straps, if needed. Skate plates may be necessary to keep the heel down.
4. Place 1-inch strips of inner tube around the footrest, covering both feet. Avoid having them too tight.
5. Place a belt midway between the upright rods of the footrest to keep legs from pushing backwards.
6. Use a thigh cuff with a tie fastened to the side of the chair for positioning. Make sure that the pull is straight out, not up or down.
7. For leg scissoring (adduction), either elevate the front of the seat cushion or insert a leg abduction pad, or do both.

## RESPONSIBILITIES FOR AND CARE OF EQUIPMENT

1. All care personnel and family members should know how the equipment is placed in the chair.
2. Care personnel and family should be taught how to position the patient properly in the wheelchair.
3. All concerned should check the individual for pressure areas and report so that alterations in positioning can be made. Checks at bath time can supplement periodic professional review.
4. Special fabric must be used for the incontinent person. Frequent cleaning and airing is necessary. Use disinfectant in solution, rinse thoroughly, and allow to dry very well. Leave various pieces apart to allow airing and drying, preferably overnight.

## CLINIC-DESIGNED REMOVABLE MODIFICATIONS

A number of inserts, clinic-designed, are available that can be added as needed and removed for convenient transport (Fig. 3-6): a seat and back support with side wings and head support; a ventilated, rolled seat (patent pending), and a footrest.

## HEAD REST

Commercially available head rests may eliminate the work of making one for the back rest. These are adjustable vertically and horizontally.

### Source

Sherfery Dentmobile, Inc.

### Construction

For those who prefer to make the insert, instructions are simple:
1. Make a waler of ¾-inch pine. It can be laid out by use of a French curve. In general, the heavier the child, the higher the curve needs to be.
2. Attach white pine slats, ⅜ inch by 1½ inches, to the formed waler, spacing the slats ¼ inch apart.
3. Attach a brace on the under side of the front edge to fit against the front cleat of the subseat.

## CLINIC-DESIGNED MODIFICATIONS FOR SMALL CHILDREN

A Tiny Tot wheelchair with clinic-designed adaptations can be an invaluable aid for a severely disabled child (Fig. 3-7A). A lapboard, whose sides are within the chair arms, may be used, so that the child's arms may extend down to reach the wheel for eventual self-wheeling. Or a utility tray, at elbow height, resting on the chair arms, can be substituted for activities or feeding (Fig. 3-7B). The value of the adaptations to provide support and security is illustrated in Figure 3-7A; this hypotonic child had never before been able to sit up.

## CLINIC-DESIGNED MODIFICATIONS FOR TEENAGERS

Other modifications, clinic-designed, can be used to meet the needs of the older, heavier disabled child (Fig. 3-8). In all cases, the adaptations should be made especially for the individual patient, as in the side supports to control and support scoliosis; the slant of the backboard and the tray (Fig. 3-8); the side wings as well as neck support; and the ankle support for the strong tension athetoid (Fig. 3-9).

**FIG. 3-7.** Tiny Tot wheelchair with rolled seat insert (patent pending), hard back with light padding, neck pillow of padded wood just below occiput, footrest with toe block, giving more freedom than ankle straps. Sides of lapbard are within chair arms so that child may reach wheels for eventual self-wheeling (*A*). Utility tray is at elbow height (*B*). Rolled, slatted seat (patent pending) and flexed footrest control extensor thrust. Safety belt is at hip bend. (Courtesy of A. Slominski, Cerebral Palsy Clinic, Indiana University Medical Center)

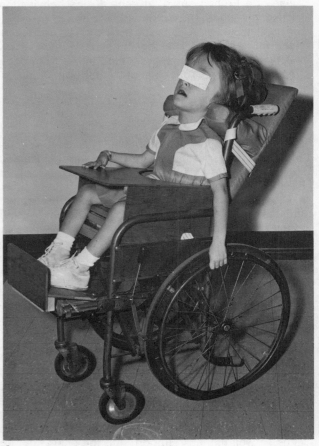

**A**

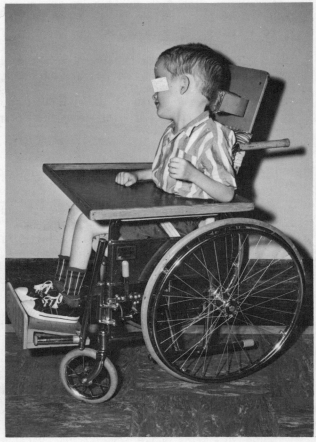

**B**

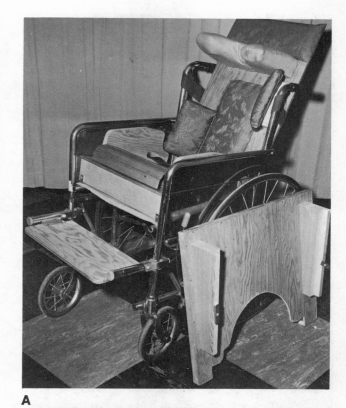

**A**

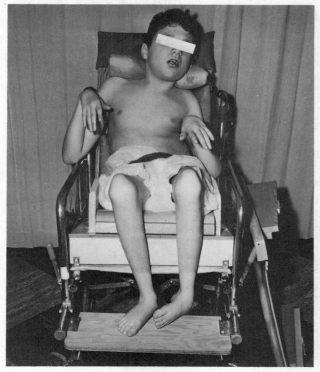

**B**

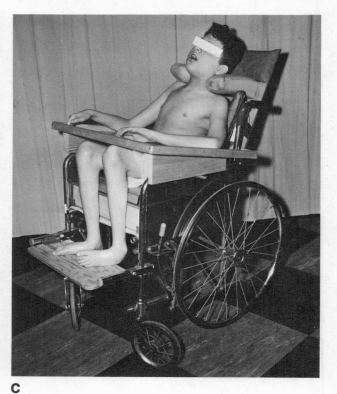

**C**

**FIG. 3-8.** Clinic-designed modifications to meet needs of older child. Side supports on backrest to support scoliosis (*A* and *B*); adjusted slant to backboard and tray (*A* and *C*). Slit in the side at the back allows seat belt to be placed in safety position. (Courtesy of A. Slominski, Cerebral Palsy Clinic, Indiana University Medical Center)

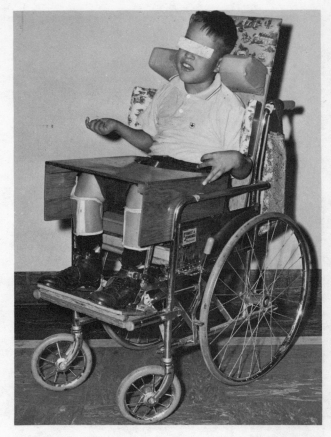

**FIG. 3-9.** Other individual adaptations for strong tension athetoid: side wings as well as neck support on backrest; and ankle support. (Courtesy of A. Slominski, Cerebral Palsy Clinic, Indiana University Medical Center)

## CLINIC-DESIGNED MODIFICATIONS FOR ADULTS

For an adult with nonfunctional ambulation (Fig. 3-10*A*), wheelchair adaptations can be introduced that will make it possible for the patient to get about. Measurements are made for proper fitting of the chair: (1) The curve of back kyphosis is measured preliminary to seat fitting; and (2) the length of the legs from hip to knees (Fig. 3-10*B*).

The wheelchair is adapted with a firm insert topped with a slatted seat insert (Fig. 3-10*C*, patent pending) to raise the knees and to prevent slouching in the leather chair; a safety belt at the hips holds the patient in place. Ankle straps are attached to the bars at each side of the footrest. The patient in Figure 3-10*C* is wearing hand and wrist splints to hold eating utensils.

A wheelchair tray can be added when needed. It is placed at elbow height, allowing the arms to rest and supporting the trunk. During meals it supports adapted feeding equipment. See section on Self-Feeding Aids for Adults in Chapter 5.

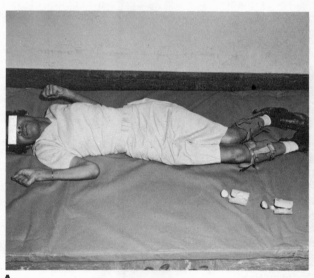

**A**

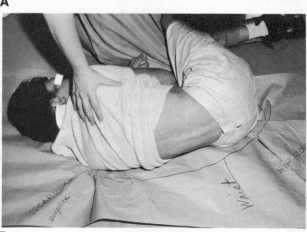

**B**

**FIG. 3-10.** Individual adaptations made for adult with non-functional ambulation (*A*), by measuring curve of kyphosis and legs from hips to knees (*B*), and adding slatted seat insert (patent pending) to lift knees, hip safety belt, and ankle straps attached to bar of footrest (*C*). (Courtesy of A. Slominski, Cerebral Palsy Clinic, Indiana University Medical Center)

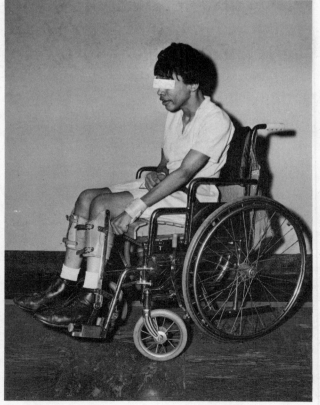

**C**

**FIG. 3-11.** Modifications to aid behavior control when lap pillow and chest restraint proved unsatisfactory (*A*). Tray, hip belt, slatted seat insert (patent pending) and chairback insert support and control body comfortably, and webbing behind legs keeps feet in place (*B*). (Courtesy of A. Slominski, Cerebral Palsy Clinic, Indiana University Medical Center)

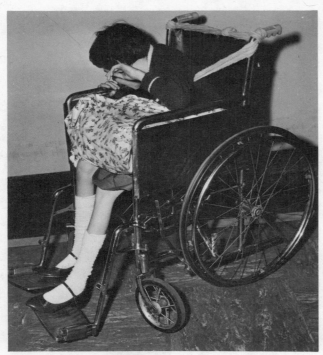

A

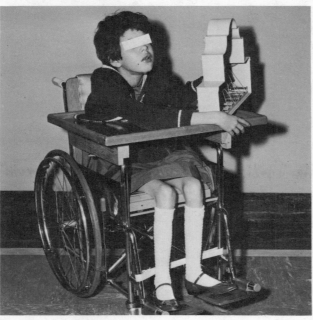

B

## CLINIC-DESIGNED MODIFICATIONS TO AID BEHAVIOR CONTROLS

Wheelchair adaptations can also be made that will aid in behavior control, as in the case of a teen-ager who was a head banger. A pillow on her lap, on which she was allowed to bang her head (Fig. 3-11*A*) proved to be an unsatisfactory solution as the chest restraint then cut into her under her armpits. When she kicked her feet, she sometimes caught them behind the footrests and was further frustrated.

Her unconstructive behavior was controlled by several adaptations: A tray fastened to the arm rests at elbow height helps keep erect posture and give arm support for handling toys placed on the tray (Fig. 3-11*B*). A seat belt at the bend of the hips is safe and comfortable but does not restrict the body. A rolled, slatted seat board insert (patent pending) and hard chairback insert keep the body from sagging in the chair. Web belting placed behind the lower legs prevents the feet from slipping back off the footrests.

## WHEELCHAIR TRAYS, FOOTRESTS, AND SEATBACKS

### WHEELCHAIR TRAY

This tray may be constructed (Fig. 3-12), but measurements must be carefully made to meet the patient's needs. The size and reach of the person for whom the tray is made, the type of activities in which he will engage, and the width of doors to be passed through will determine the dimensions of the tray. The average tray board for adults is 23 by 26 inches; for children, 16 by 21 inches.

### Construction

1. Measure for size of tray. Measure for width and depth of cutout (Fig. 3-12, *E-H-G*). It must fit the individual; the back edges of the tray (Fig. 3-12, *AG* and *ED*) should be flush with back upright of wheelchair. For depth (Fig. 3-12, *FH*), measure back to front of body at level of flexed elbows. For width (*GE*), measure left side of the trunk to right side. If the patient wears braces, make measurements with braces on. Allow 1 inch extra for winter clothes. For the comfort of a person with scoliosis, the opening may need to be cut off-center, to right or to left.
2. Measure for height of tray. Flex the elbow at 90

degrees and place the forearm and hands on tray. If the tray does not rest on the wheelchair arms when the individual is in this position, measure the distance from the underside of the tray to the place where board will rest on the arm of the chair or be attached to the chair arm. This measurement will vary according to the method selected for fastening the tray. If the tray is properly fitted, the individual cannot get his arms down through the cutout space of the tray. This maintains posture and provides safety from falling. See Posture Pointers above.

3. For the tray, use ⅜-inch good quality plywood or Masonite with Formica for the top surface. For the supports (*J*), use wood blocks approximately 11 inches long. See Methods of Fastening Tray for different widths and depths, as needed. For the rail or edging, use screen molding R or hardwood stripping (white pine). Glue, nails, and epoxy varnish or Minowax will also be needed, the latter to protect the wood and plywood.
4. Cut the tray to the dimensions determined.
5. Sand all surfaces of plywood.
6. Glue and nail molding, using 1-inch wire brads, to the top of the board with the straight edge inside; or glue and nail wooden strips to the outside edge of the board.
7. Finish with varnish after supports or tray raisers, if needed, are added.

## Tray Raisers

Two blocks of wood about 11 inches long can be cut at the height needed to position the arms as described above (Fig. 3-13). If necessary, the blocks also can be graduated to give slope to the tray (see Fig. 3-8*C*). The width of raiser blocks will depend upon whether they will be the only item between the bottom of the tray and the arms of the wheelchair or whether they will be part of the supports which fasten the tray to the arm of the wheelchair.

## Methods for Fastening Tray to Unupholstered Arm

The tray may be fastened to chair arms that have no upholstery by one of the following methods:
1. Attach tray near the back edges (Fig. 3-12, *AG* and *ED* at position I). This method can be used alone only when the individual using the chair is coordinated and has little tension or extraneous motion. Other methods are stronger.
2. One alternative to the above method is to drill holes

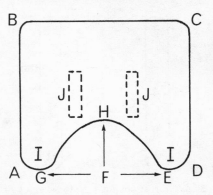

**FIG. 3-12.** Diagram for constructing wheelchair tray. *A-B* and *B-C,* outside dimensions; *A-G* and *E-D,* width of extenders at back edge; *FH,* depth of cutout; *GE,* width of cutout; *I,* position for one method of attachment to wheelchair without upholstered arms; *J,* position for blocks on underside of tray for attachment to chair with upholstered arms. (Courtesy of staff of Indiana University Medical Center and staff of Warren G. Murray Children's Center, Centralia, Ill.)

**FIG. 3-13.** Tray-raisers to fit arms of wheelchair. (Courtesy of staff of Indiana University Medical Center and staff of Warren G. Murray Children's Center, Centralia, Ill.)

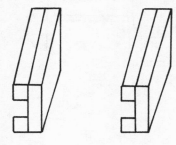

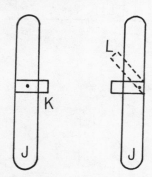

**FIG. 3-14.** Blocks for attaching tray to wheelchair with upholstered arms, positioned at point *J* in Figure 3-12. *K,* permanent metal fastener; *L,* rotating metal fastener. (Courtesy of staff of Indiana University Medical Center and staff of Warren G. Murray Children's Center, Centralia, Ill.)

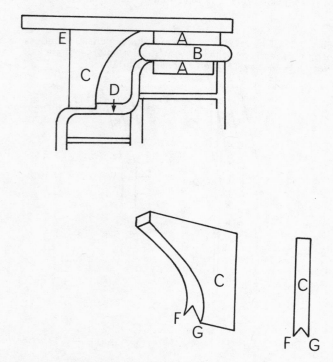

**FIG. 3-15.** Diagram for constructing tray for wheelchair with desk arms. *At left,* side view shows provimal supports, *A,* going above and below armrests, *B;* distal support, *C,* resting on lower extension of chair arm, *D;* bottom of tray, *E. At right,* side and front views of distal support, *C,* showing notch, *FG* to fit on chair arm. (Courtesy of the staff of Indiana Medical Center and the staff of the Warren G. Murray Children's Center, Centralia, Ill.)

at least 1 inch in from the ends. Cloth straps or round plastic belts can be drawn through holes and tied around the back of the chair.

3. Another alternative is to fasten the ends of seat belts by panel cement or wood staples to edges *AG* and *ED* and buckle the belt behind the chair.

4. A fourth method is to place sliding bolt locks on the tray extenders, near back edges (see Fig. 3-17).

5. Screw four tool holders (medium size, made by Masonite Corp.) to bottom of tray in such a position as to allow two to clip onto each arm of the chair, gripping at the back and at the front. Check the size of the tool-holder clip to be sure it grips the wheelchair arm before fastening it to the tray. These clips cannot be relied upon for young children, nor should they be the only grippers for the tray for persons with strong uncontrolled motion.

6. Use a draw catch with safety snap (a wire spring snap) to keep the tray in place and to guard against opening. For persons with severe involuntary motion, two draw catches have been used on each side (see Figure 3-16). Notice that the support for the fasteners consists of three parts: the tray raiser section from the undersurface to tray to the top of the arm (see also Figure 3-13); a connecting unit which is screwed to the raiser and to the under block; and the block which fits under the chair arm and is screwed to the connecting unit. These three-part supports are attached to the tray so that the opening of each faces the same way. Therefore, one will grip one wheelchair arm from its *outer* surface. The other will grip the other wheelchair arm from the *inner* surface, making it possible to attach the draw catch with safety snap on the outside surface of this wheelchair arm.

### Methods of Fastening Tray to Upholstered Arms

The following methods may be used to supplement techniques described in the foregoing section.

1. Cut two hardwood blocks, approximately 11 inches by 1½ inches by 1⅛ inches. The ends of the blocks may be rounded. When the tray is set on the wheelchair arms, these blocks will fit at approximately the position shown in Figure 3-12, *J,* on the underside of the tray. In this position, they will be just *outside* the arms of the wheelchair. Mark position with a pencil on the underside of the tray. Glue and nail the blocks into position, and varnish the tray and blocks. When dry, screw one permanent metal fastener (*K*) at midpoint of one block and one rotating metal fastener (*L*) at mid-

point of the other block (Fig. 3-14). To ensure greater security and to prevent the tray from pushing away from the body, use four metal fasteners: one of each set may be placed at about 2 inches from each end of the supporting block. The two rotating fasteners will be on the same block.

2. Use Lap Tray Fastener Kit (see Figure 3-18) distributed by Fred Sammons, Inc.

3. See utility tray in Figure 3-3 for positioning of elastic cords and no-slip pads which make reliable and easy fasteners.

## TRAY FOR WHEELCHAIR WITH DESK ARMS

A board for this tray (Fig. 3-15) can be shaped as the one shown in Figure 3-12. The method of measuring should be the same. Proximal supports (*A*), in the diagram at the left, which hold the tray fasteners, and any raisers that may be needed must be made *shorter* than the armrests (*B*)

For the distal supports (*C*), which rest on the lower extension of the chair arm (*D*), use two pieces of hardwood about 1¼ inches thick. These should be cut 4½ inches wide. The length will depend upon the distance from the bottom of the tray (*E*) to the top of the lower extension (*D*), plus 1 inch. The lower edge of the distal support can be notched, as shown in diagram at right in Figure 3-15, to hold it firmly on the lower extension bar of the chair arm.

## TRAY FOR COLSON WHEELCHAIR

The Warren G. Murray Children's Center, Centralia, Ill., purchases Colson chairs without seats or footrests, adds Everest & Jennings footrests, and builds parts to give individualized fit and function (Fig. 3-16). Notice the backboard, and notice also that the tray is held on the left arm of the chair in such a way that the arm of the wheelchair is gripped from its *outer* side. The tray is held in place by wood placed just *inside* the right arm (see also Figure 3-13). Draw catches with safety snaps are attached to this wooden support.

## FASTENERS FOR COMMERCIAL TRAYS

The Adjusto Tray (Everest & Jennings, Inc. J 2044) and the Maple Lap Tray of Fred Sammons, Inc. may be modified for better function. As purchased, the tray cutouts are too shallow and do not project far enough back. The cutout may be shaped and deepened by adding wooden extenders so that the tray assumes the functional shape necessary to fit the

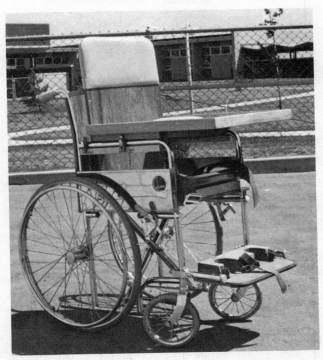

**FIG. 3-16.** Colson wheelchair with specially made seat, backboard, and tray for individualized fit. Of particular interest is the method of fastening tray to chair arms. (Courtesy of the Illinois Department of Mental Health, Warren G. Murray Children's Center, Centralia, Ill.)

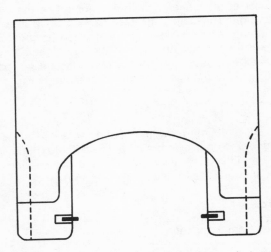

**FIG. 3-17.** Diagram of extender that may be made to adjust size of cutout on tray. Bolts will hold tray to back uprights of chair. (Courtesy of P. Holser Buehler, Los Angeles County Development Center and Don Guetti, Everest & Jennings, Inc.)

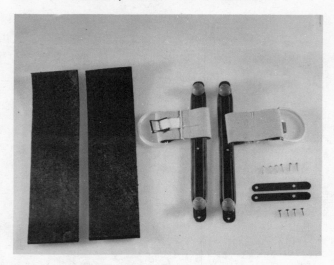

**FIG. 3-18.** Lap tray fastener kit, containing sponge rubber with peel-off backing, to attach to tray bottom; bars with rubber belt that will hold tray; side brackets; and the screws to attach bars and brackets to tray. (Courtesy of Fred Sammons, Inc., Brookfield, Ill.)

individual user. Indent the outer edges, near the back of the tray and extenders (Fig. 3-17) to permit the user to reach the wheels of his chair easily.

Sliding bolt locks may be added near the end of each extender to fasten the tray to the back uprights of the wheelchair. Holes must be drilled in the back uprights of the wheelchair to accommodate the bolts. When bolted in place, the tray cannot move forward. Additional fasteners may be used, such as those described for the construction of the wheelchair tray, if required by heavy duty. A rim may also be added to the tray to keep items from rolling or sliding off.

## LAP TRAY FASTENER KIT

A kit containing parts needed to add Sure-Grip Fasteners to your own lap trays is available (Fig. 3-18). It is simplified for easy assembly and comes with detailed instructions for use.

### Source

Fred Sammons, Inc.

## FOOTREST FOR COLSON WHEELCHAIR

A footrest that will firmly hold the feet in place is constructed of ½-inch plywood with a heel guide of

2- by 4-inch pine (see Figure 3-16). The openings in the heel guide are cut large enough to accept the heel and back of the individual's shoes. Straps hold the feet in place. The spacing between the cutouts will be determined by the width that is comfortable for the person using the chair.

## SHOE ATTACHMENT FOR PUSHING

A device designed for severely disabled young adults who are wheelchair-bound provides a means by which they may move the chair themselves (Fig. 3-19). However, the only method of locomotion is to push the chair backwards with one foot. The device can also be used as a brake when the chair is moving forward down gentle slopes.

### Construction

1. A crutch tip is put onto a piece of steel pipe of a length cut to the individual's need.
2. The other end of the pipe is soldered to a metal plate, which is then riveted to the shoe. Be sure that the rivets are not in a position to irritate the foot.
3. A hightop shoe may be needed for extra support to the ankle in pushing.

**FIG. 3-19.** Shoe attachment worn by wheelchair patient to move the chair or to stop it. (Courtesy of N. S. Greenberg, Department of Rehabilitation Medicine, Bird S. Coler Hospital, New York, N.Y.)

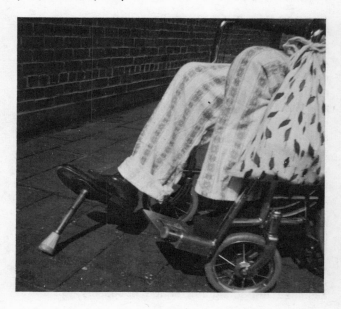

## WHEELCHAIR NARROWING BAR

A bar can be made that will reduce the width of a folding wheelchair, making it possible to negotiate narrow doorways or passages (Fig. 3-20). For emergency purposes, a wire coat hanger looped around the pushing handles will suffice. A commercial product is also available.

### Source

Everest & Jennings, Inc.

### CONSTRUCTION

1. Use cold-rolled steel, ¼ inch by 1 inch.
2. The easiest way to measure for the length of the bar is to collapse the wheelchair and place it in the narrowest door opening to be used. Then open the chair to within practical limits for passage through the doorway and measure from the outside horizontal limits of the wheelchair frame for the length needed.
3. Bend tabs (*A-B* and *C-D*) at 90 degrees. The vertical tabs should be no longer than 1 inch or 1¼ inch.
4. Wrap the entire bar with rubberized tape to prevent slipping.
5. Apply bar over wheelchair frame to hold it in narrowed position.
6. If the chair seat sags, put in a seatboard.

### PADDED SEATBOARD

A comfortable padded seatboard can be made for a wheelchair (Fig. 3-21).

### Construction

1. All measurements are taken of the patient in the prone position on a *firm* surface.
2. Place a ruler between the legs, perpendicular to the bed at the crotch. Measure from the bed to the height of the end of the spine and add 4 inches (Fig. 3-21,*a*).
3. Find the widest distance between the bones that the patient sits on and add 2 inches to this measurement (Fig. 3-21,*b*).
4. Cut a piece of ⅝-inch plywood board to fit over the seat of the wheelchair, but not so wide as to obstruct removal of the chair arms (if they are removable).

5. At the center back of the board (*DC*), make a semicircular cutout the depth of *a* and the width of *b*.
6. Add a foam rubber pad 3 inches thick that measures *AB* by *BC*. No cutout should be made in this. Cover with washable material.

## WHEELCHAIR SAFETY BELTS AND SUPPORTS

### JIFFY RESTRAINT FOR YOUNG ADULTS

The Jiffy Restraint is made of webbing with a Velcro fastening. Care must be taken not to fasten the belt so that it grips around the stomach or chest. Bring the belt up from seat level and the back of the seat, as in auto safety belts.

### Sources

Fred Sammons, Inc.
Smalley & Bates, Inc.

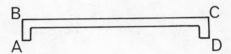

**FIG. 3-20.** Wheelchair narrowing bar. *B-C,* width of bar; *A* and *D,* vertical tabs. (Courtesy of B. Crowder and United Cerebral Palsy of Pennsylvania)

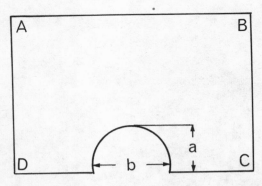

**FIG. 3-21.** Diagram for constructing seatboard for wheelchair. *A-B* and *B-C,* dimensions of board; *a,* depth as measured from bed surface to end of spine, plus 4 inches; *b,* width of distance between patient's "seat bones," plus 2 inches. (Courtesy of the Institute of Rehabilitation Medicine, New York University Medical Center)

## PERMA-SAFE BELT

This belt safeguards against accidental falls. The model features back adjustments that are out of the patient's reach (Fig. 3-22). It is available in various colors of 2-inch cotton or nylon webbing.

### Source

Shelton Industries

## SAFETY BELT WITH AIRCRAFT TYPE BUCKLE

Sports shops, Scouts shops, and the companies whose catalogs are listed in the Reference section of this chapter have this belt available.

## ARMY OR SCOUT WEB BELTS WITH FLAT BUCKLES

An easily available belt, this one can serve many needs. On the wheelchair, the belt can be looped under the seat and drawn up between the seat and side, near the back, in a position similar to that of auto or airplane safety seat belts. The width depends on the size of the patient, since support with freedom from chafing is the objective.

# VEHICLE ADAPTATIONS TO ACCOMMODATE WHEELCHAIRS

### General Considerations

A bus should not be too large to be maneuvered through narrow, crowded streets.

From the standpoint of loading and unloading, a wide right-side entrance affords convenience and safety (Fig. 3-23). An emergency rear door provides a third point of access.

Safety belts should be attached to seats for every passenger, and the wheelchairs themselves should be kept from rolling in the bus by floor fasteners provided for each chair.

A hydraulic lift for wheelchair occupants is a practical addition.

### Precautions

1. Wheelchair seat belts should be closed during lift and during transport.
2. Ramps and self-storing ramps should be securely fitted when in use.
3. Wheelchairs should be brought down the ramp *backward,* with the large wheels leading.

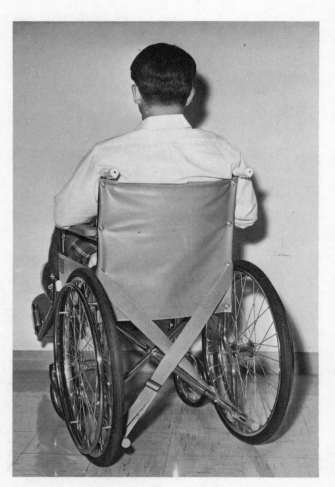

**FIG. 3-22.** Perma-Safe seat belt, with adjustments at back, out of patient's reach. (Courtesy of Shelton Industries, Midway City, Calif.)

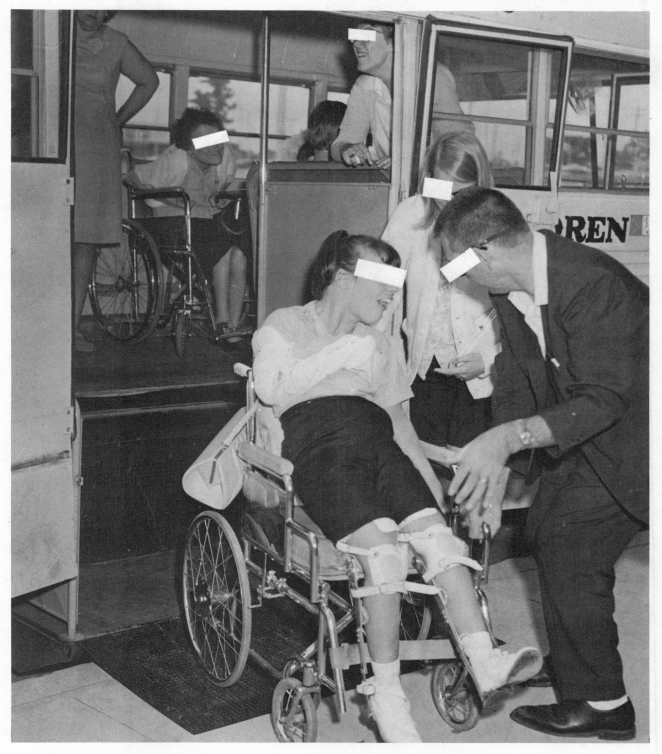

**FIG. 3-23.** Wide side door of bus, facilitating loading and unloading of wheelchairs. (Courtesy of United Cerebral Palsy of Ohio)

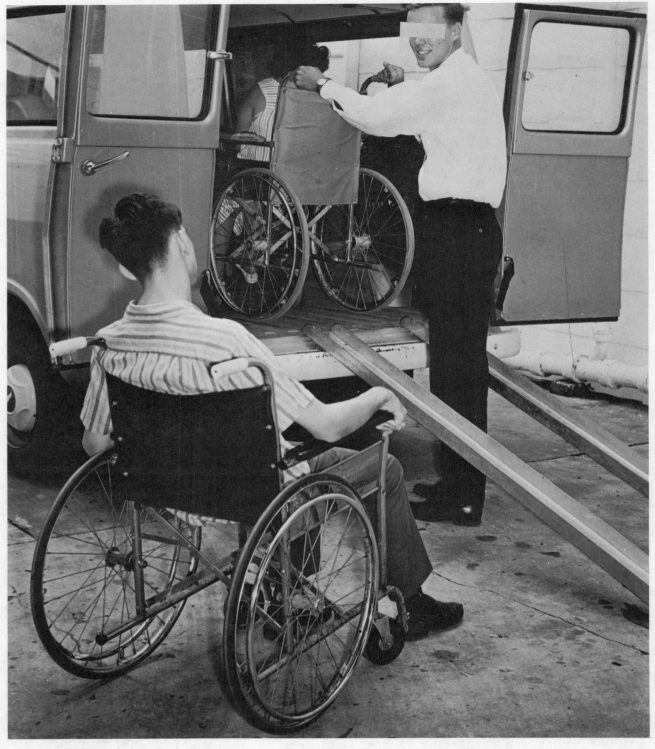

**FIG. 3-24.** Back-door ramp for use with Minibus. Easily constructed, it hooks onto rear bumper. Chairs should be brought down backwards for safety. (Courtesy of J.Bresnahan and P. White, United Cerebral Palsy of New Orleans, Inc.)

## COMMERICAL RAMPS AND VEHICLE LOADING DEVICES

Several companies manufacture and distribute ramps and vehicle-loading equipment.

### Sources

Copperloy Corp. (Telescope Wheelchair Ramp)
Handi-Ramp Inc.
Nelson Enterprises (Porta-Ramp Wheelchair Carrier)

## COMMERCIAL ADAPTATIONS

The United Cerebral Palsy Association of King County, Washington, has a bus adapted to haul 18 persons, plus driver and helper. Ten passengers remain in wheelchairs, and eight are placed in seats around the perimeter of the cab and fastened in with seat belts.

### Sources

Allied Body Works, Inc.
Franklin Body and Equipment Corp.
Sheller-Globe, Superior Southern Division and Superior Coach Division

## COMMERCIALLY AVAILABLE SPECIAL TRANSPORTATION VEHICLES

Wheelchairs may be folded and placed within a car or on an auto rack. However, several types of special vehicles are manufactured for transporting wheelchairs.

### Sources

Checker Motor Sales Corporation (Standard Wheelchair Sedan; Raised-Roof Wheelchair Sedan that accommodates passenger sitting in regular or electric wheelchair models; Marathon Wheelchair Limousine that holds up to three vehicles)
Minibus, Inc. (Minibus that accommodates 10 wheelchairs and 6 seated passengers or five wheelchairs and 19 seated; front wheel drive with lower floor)

## WHEELCHAIR RAMP FOR MINIBUS

Ramps can be constructed for both a rear door and a side door (Figs. 3-24 and 3-25) of a Minibus or other transportation vehicle. It is advisable to have a local sheet metal shop do the work.

### Construction of Back Door Ramp

1. Ramps should measure 6 feet in length and 5 inches wide. Sides should be 2 inches high.
2. A cross piece of the same material is attached to the ramps at approximately a 45-degree angle. This piece is made to hook onto the rear bumper.
3. The cross piece, which rests between the bumper and the vehicle must be attached to the ramp in a location that will allow the top of the ramp to rest level and to fit flush with the floor of the vehicle.
4. Wheelchair is brought down backwards for safety.

### Construction of Side Door Ramp

1. Make ramps (Fig. 3-25) 2 inches shorter than vehicle's inside width so they may be stored crosswise inside.
2. Channel (*C*) should be 5 inches wide, with sides 2 inches high.
3. At the end of the channel that will hook (*H*) onto the vehicle, bend 2½ inches of the ramp down to form a 25-degree angle.
4. Ramp is held to door sill (*S*) of vehicle by two 1-inch diameter pins (flathead stove bolts). These should project at least ⅝ inch and can be used as bolts turned into holes tapped in the channel (*C*), placed 3 inches apart.
5. The pins fit into anchor holes placed 3 inches apart in the body.

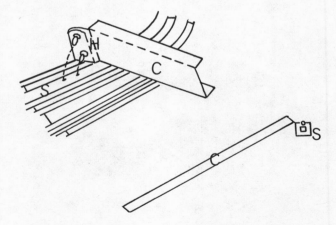

**FIG. 3-25.** Diagram for construction of side-door ramp for Minibus. *At left,* underside view of ramp channel, *C,* showing method of attachment by bolts, *H,* to doorsill, *S,* of bus. *At right,* side view of ramp, *C,* showing bend made to fit onto door sill, *S,* with bolts. (Courtesy of J. Bresnahan and P. White, United Cerebral Palsy of New Orleans, Inc.)

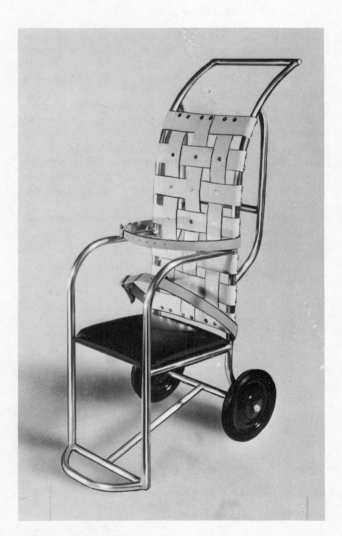

**FIG. 3-26.** Hogg chair, useful for short-term use—from one room to another. (Courtesy of Hogg Chair Co., Chicago Ill.)

## HOGG CHAIR

This chair comes in three sizes for ages 3 to 11 years (Fig. 3-26).

### Source

Hogg Chair Co.

### Precautions

1. Do not use for long periods of sitting, although the chair is efficient for transferring the patient short distances. Some athetoid children are disturbed by being tipped back when pushed.
2. Use a seat belt, not a top strap. Substitute auto type diagonal webbing for the top strap.

## SUFFOLK MULTIPURPOSE CHAIR-TABLE

For multiply handicapped children, this chair features a removable swing-away, self-storing table. The chair has an adjustable headrest, an adjustable, oversize, one-piece footrest, and a front-to-back adjustable seat that can be angled for better positioning. It is mounted on casters and wheels with anti-tipping legs.

### Source

Lumex, Inc.

## MOBILE LOUNGE

Made for adults only, this mobile chair (Fig. 3-27) has a multiposition tray that snaps on and off and is stored at the side of the chair. The chair has a foam-padded back, seat, and armrests, covered with vinyl. There are other models of similar design.

### Sources

Everest & Jennings, Inc.
G. E. Miller, Inc.
J. A. Preston Corp.
Sears Roebuck local stores or write Medical Division

## ECONOMY WHEELCHAIR (STARLINER)

An economy wheelchair line called "Starliner" is adequate for use during outdoor recreation—on a lawn or at the beach.

**Source**

Everest & Jennings, Inc.

# MECHANICAL LIFTS FOR THE PATIENT

### HYDRAULIC PATIENT LIFTER PC 7183

This device permits moving a patient to and from a wheelchair, bed, exercise mat, toilet, easy chair, or car (Fig. 3-28). A slight person—nurse or attendant—can lift and transfer a heavy patient with ease and safety.

The lift can be stored under a bed or in a car trunk. It has a standard U base, 5-inch casters, and a canvas seat and backrest (nylon also available). The capacity is 450 pounds.

The same lift with an adjustable U base (PC 7183C) can be adjusted to pass through a 24-inch doorway.

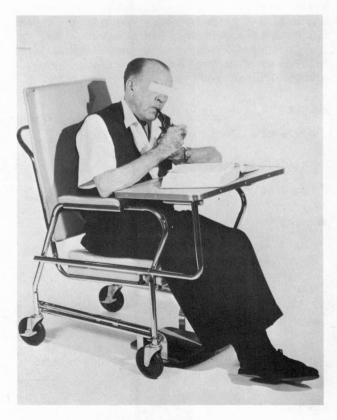

**FIG. 3-27.** Mobile lounge chair, suitable for adults only. (Courtesy of Everest & Jennings, Inc., Los Angeles, Calif.)

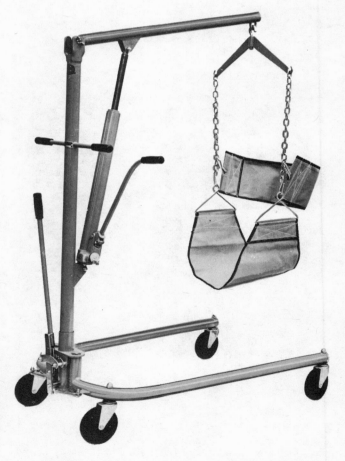

**FIG. 3-28.** Hydraulic Patient Lifter PC 7183, that permits easy and safe transfer of patient by one person. (Copyright 1965 by J. A. Preston Corporation)

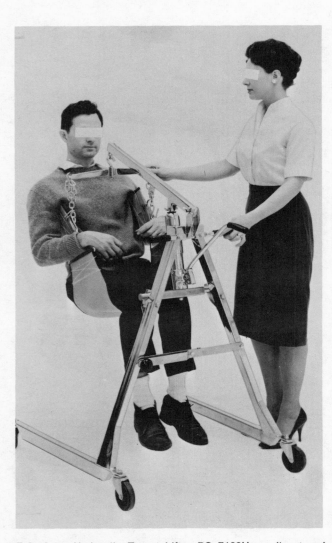

**FIG. 3-29.** Hydraulic Travel Lifter PC 7189H, easily stored in car trunk for convenient use on trips. It is not intended for severely disabled patient. (Copyright 1965 by J. A. Preston Corporation)

### Source

J. A. Preston Corp.

### HYDRAULIC TRAVEL LIFTER PC 7189H

This lift is designed specifically for travel (Fig. 3-29). Its unique folding feature simplifies handling and easy storage in a car trunk. It is not intended for the severely involved patient or one who may require head support.

### Source

J. A. Preston Corp.

### KARTOP LIFT PC 7187

The lift mounts on top of the car and enables the attendant to lift the disabled patient out of his wheelchair and place him in the seat with almost no effort at all. The Kartop rests on sturdy rubber suction cups and is held in place by hooks that snap under the drip eave. It is adjustable to cars of various widths. No change is made on the car itself—no holes drilled, no brackets attached. The lift remains in place on the car top; the lifting arm slides out, ready for instant use.

### Source

J. A. Preston Corp.

### SWIMMING POOL LIFT

Lifts are also available for use at poolside.

### Sources

Ted Hoyer & Co., Inc.
G. E. Miller, Inc.
J. A. Preston Corp.
Trans-Aid Corp.

### MARK II TRANSVERSE LIFT

This lift moves easily through any door or passageway. Its unique transverse base eliminates adjustments for narrow openings (Fig. 3-30).

### Source

Trans-Aid Corp.

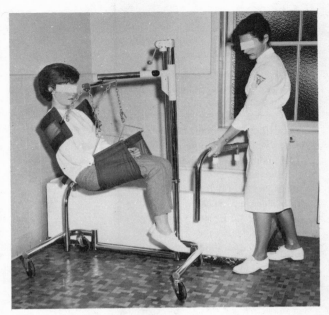

**FIG. 3-30.** Mark II Transverse Lift, easily maneuvered through narrow doors and passageways. (Courtesy of Trans-Aid Corp., Inglewood, Calif.)

## E-Z BATH LIFT

This lift is useful at home if the top is adjusted to hold the patient with cerebral palsy in it.

### Source

Eaton E-Z Bath Co.

## SLIDING ARM WHEELCHAIR LOADER

An electrically operated hoist on this loader helps the attendant to place the patient in a wheelchair.

### Source

Robin-Aids, Inc.

## THE WHEEL-O-VATOR

This elevator is designed specifically for unassisted use by someone in a wheelchair (Fig. 3-31).

### Source

Wheelchair Elevators, Inc.

### Specifications

The elevator has a maximum lifting height of 5 feet and a minimum of 2 inches. The motor operates on ¾ horsepower, 110 volts AC (household current). It must be set down on a flat surface. Other than consideration of porch height (maximum 5 feet), no further installation or adjustment is required.

The unit is constructed of cold-rolled square steel tubing, finished in lacquer, either black or gray. Gates are optional and must be ordered with the machine. The elevator is designed for long life against weather and wear and requires only minor maintenance.

### Manufacturer's Claims

According to the manufacturer's description, the elevator's purpose is to take the place of dangerous ramps and to make it possible for a person in a wheelchair to come and go without having to have help. All that is necessary is to push the switch for "up" or "down."

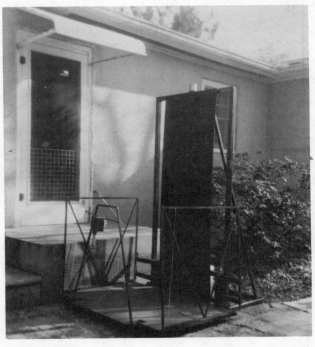

**FIG. 3-31.** The Wheel-O-Vator, with maximum lift of 5 feet, intended for use without assistance simply by pushing on-off switch. (Courtesy of Wheelchair Elevators, Inc., Broussard, La.)

### Other Elevators and Their Sources

(All designed essentially for home installation)
"Elevette": Inclinator Company of America
"Escalift": Dover Corp.
"Inclinator-Elevette": Inclinator-Elevette Co.
"Residence Elevator": G. E. Miller, Inc.
"Stair Glide": G. E. Miller, Inc.

## ARCHITECTURAL BARRIERS TO SELF-HELP

Wheelchair users and their families are well aware that few buildings are constructed to accommodate a wheelchair. There are numerous sources of information on the subject, listed in the References section of this chapter.

## REFERENCES

### Evaluation, Maintenance, and Use of Wheelchairs

Brent, S. "Basic considerations in prescribing wheelchairs," Am J Phys Med 39:47, 1960.

Coll, L. "Thirteen years ago I bought a wheelchair," The Apothecary, Oct., p. 30, 1963.

Deaver, G., Brittis, A. *Braces, Crutches and Wheelchairs.* New York, New York University Medical Center, 1953.

Fahland, B., Grendahl, B. *Wheelchair Selection: More Than Choosing A Chair With Wheels.* Minneapolis, American Rehabilitation Foundation Publications Office, 1967. (Appendix includes plans for a sliding board, lapboards, seatboard, and ramp.)

Fowles, B. H. "Evaluation and selection of wheelchairs," Phys Ther Rev 39:525, 1959. (Free reprint: Highland View Hospital.)

Goss, J. "Sickroom basics, wheelchairs and walkers," Rental Equipment Register, Nov. 1963.

Guttman, L. "A symposium on the wheelchair," Paraplegia News 11:20, 1964.

Hoberman, M., Cicenia, E., Sampson, O. "Maintenance and minor repairs of the wheelchair," Am J Phys Med 35:206, 1956.

Lawton, E. *Activities of Daily Living.* New York, McGraw-Hill, 1962.

Lowman, E., Rusk, H. "Selection of Wheelchairs," *Self-Help Devices,* Part 1, Rehab Mono 21, 1962.

Peizer, E., Wright, D., Freiberger, H. "Bioengineering methods of wheelchair evaluation," Bull Prosth Res 10:77, 1964.

Rayner, C. Wheelchairs, Design 164:30, 1962.

"Report on a conference for wheelchair manufacturers," Bull Prosth Res Spring, 1965. (Also available from Superintendent of Documents, U.S. Government Printing Office, Washington, D.C. 20402, 70 cents)

Rullstolar. *Information for Vanforevarden,* Bromma, Sweden. ICTA Information Centre, 1964.

"Self-elevating wheelchair," Lancet 1:1306, 1964.

"Wheelchair Prescription," PHS Rehabilitation Guide, Series I, No. 1666. Superintendent of Documents, Washington, D.C.

"Wheelchairs," Rehabilitation Gazett 9:76, 1966.

### Catalogs of Manufacturers and Distributors of Wheelchairs

American Wheelchair, Cincinnati, Ohio.

Colson Co., Chicago, Ill.

Dawson, Milburn & Co., Torquay, Devon, England

Everest & Jennings, Inc., Los Angeles, Calif.

Hogg Chair Co., Chicago, Ill.

ICTA Information Centre, Bromma 3, Sweden

The Kendall Co., Hospital Products Division, Chicago, Ill.

Lumex, Inc., Bay Shore, N.Y.

G. E. Miller, Inc., Yonkers, N.Y.

J. A. Preston Corp., New York, N.Y.

Rehab Aids, Miami, Fla.

Stainless Medical Products, Santa Ana, Calif.

### Catalogs of Manufacturers and Distributors of Power-Driven Wheelchairs

Orthopedia-GMBH, Salzreder, Germany. (Electro Folding Chair)

American Wheel Chair Co., Cincinnati, Ohio. (Electromatic)

Grewe & Shulte-Derne, Derner Strasse, Germany (Elkamobile)

Laminex, Inc., Maple Plain, Minn.

Moonwalker of Space General Company, El Monte, Calif.

Everest & Jennings, Los Angeles, Calif. (Motorized Wheel Chair)

MEYRA Wheelchairs Factory, Germany. (Uni-Stair Climbing Wheelchair and Electromobile "Movra")

### Architectural Barriers That Hinder the Physically Handicapped

"American Standards Association Specifications for Making Building and Facilities Accessible to, and Usable by, the Physically Handicapped," National Easter Seal Society for Crippled Children and Adults, Inc., 1961.

"Building Standards for the Handicapped—National Building Code of Canada," Associate Committee on the National Building Code, Suppl. 7 NRC No. 8333, National Research Council, 1965.

"Directions for the Preparation of a Guide for Disabled Persons in Towns and other Built-up Areas," International Information Centre on Technical Aids, International Society for Rehabilitation of the Disabled.

"Breaking Down the Architectural Barriers," The President's Committee on Employment of the Physically Handicapped, 1965.

"Facilities in Public Buildings for Persons with Ambulatory Impairments," U.S. Department of Labor, 1958.

Goldsmith, S. *Designing for the Disabled.* London, Royal Institute of British Architects, Technical Information Service, 1963.

"Instructions to Architects on Provisions for the Handicapped," Facilities Planning Division, New York State Department of Mental Hygiene, 1964.

*Interim Guide: Performance Criteria on Spatial Organization for the Physically Handicapped,* Albany State University Construction Fund, 1965.

*Making Facilities Accessible to the Physically Handicapped,* Albany State University Construction Fund, 1966.

Nugent, T. J. "Design of buildings to permit their use by the handicapped," New Building Research, Fall: 51, 1960.

"A Plan for the Living Accommodation of the Adult Cerebral Palsied," Spastic Center of New South Wales, 1968.

"Program of Requirements for a School for the Severely Handicapped," Human Resources Center, Educational Research Services, 1963.

Salmon, F. C., Salmon, C. F. *Rehabilitation Center Planning.* University Park, Pa., Pennsylvania State Univ. Press, 1959.

Yuker, H. E., Cohen, A., Feldman, M. A. "The Development and Effects of an Inexpensive Elevator for Eliminating Architectural Barriers in Public Buildings," Projected Report RD-1651-G VRA, Hofstra Univ., 1966.

# 4

# Lifting, Carrying, and Transfer

This chapter will replace the UCP booklet *Parent Series Aid: Assisting the Cerebral Palsied Child: Lifting and Carrying.* Many pointers in the original booklet are still useful and will be repeated. However, the present philosophy of rehabilitation would require the title to be changed to *Assisting the Handicapped Child To Move: Transfer Activities.* He is no longer considered a passive weight to be lifted and carried; his cooperation is required whenever possible. He frequently has a wheelchair to which he is transferred rather than lifted, and devices within the means of families and clinics are now available for passive lifting so that parents and therapists can preserve their backs and their energies for other tasks. Therefore, this section will outline how adults can best control their own body mechanics when helping a handicapped child and will describe what mechanical aids exist to ease their efforts. (See also the section on Mechanical Lifts for Patients in Chapter 3 and the section on Bathing Equipment in Chapter 7.)

## LIFTING

The general principles of lifting, lowering, carrying, and transferring (Fig. 4-1) apply whether one is lifting a wheelchair into a car trunk or transferring a nonweightbearing child into another conveyance. Step-by-step procedures in all situations are as follows.

1. Understand that general principles are always the same, but the easiest method varies with the capabilities of the helper, as well as those of the patient.
2. Find out how much the cerebral palsied individual is accustomed to doing for himself.
3. Determine how much he can cooperate in the proposed change of position.
4. Have him take part in every change of position as much as possible.
5. Assist him to move with as little lifting, carrying, or lowering on your part as possible; use a mechanical aid whenever possible.

### PRINCIPLES OF GOOD LIFTING

1. First plan the job.
2. Be sure that there is ample room for good footing and that the path is cleared for the carry or transfer.
3. Stand so you will not have to twist your body as you lift the patient.
4. Stand close to the load, with one foot ahead of the other; the foot that is ahead should usually be in the direction you are going (Fig. 4-2).
5. Do not try to lift from a kneeling position, as this takes away the power source. However, with smaller children or loads, it may be advantageous to start to lift with one knee on the floor.
6. Get a good grasp before starting to lift.
7. Make a preliminary heft to see if the load is within your capacity.
8. If the weight of the load is more than one-fourth of your body weight or if it is awkward, you should get someone to help you.
9. Lift one end of the load slightly, if necessary, so you can place one hand underneath it in order to get a firm grasp.
10. Get your legs ready for the lift by bending them. Do not attempt to lift a load with your legs bent beyond a right-angle position.
11. Lower your body near the level of the object to be lifted.
12. Be sure your back is straight. If it is neither

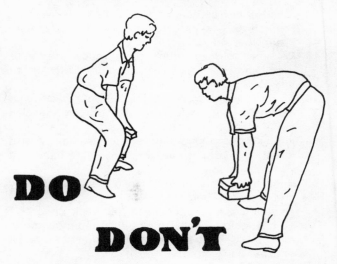

**FIG. 4-1.** Correct method of lifting (*left*) and incorrect (*right*). Keep the back as straight as possible and bend the knees; lift by straightening the knees. Do not keep the legs rigid and bend from the waist or severe back strain may result. (From Assisting the Cerebral Palsied Child: Lifting and Carrying. Reproduced with permission)

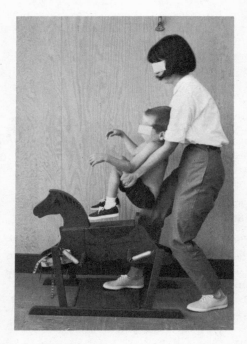

**FIG. 4-2.** Lifting child onto rocking horse. One foot is placed ahead of the other, in the direction of the move. (From Svirsky, H. S. The severely involved child: Maternal backache. *Clin Orthop 47:*59, 1966. Reproduced with permission)

rounded nor arched, and is as near the vertical position as possible, you will avoid strain. Also, "keep your shirt loose."

13. Be sure your shoulders are directly over your knees and your hands reach straight downward to the load.
14. To be in the proper position, let your back muscles hold your back steady as your leg muscles get ready to go to work.
15. Lift by straightening your legs in a steady upward thrust, and at the same time move your back to a vertical position.
16. Keep the weight of the load close to your body and over your feet.
17. As your legs straighten, keep your back straight.
18. To change direction during a lift, step around and turn your whole body, without twisting at the waist or lower back.

## DRAWING HEAVY CHILD TO NEAR SIDE OF BED

1. Stand close to the bed with one leg forward and weight over it.
2. Sink with knees bent to a crouch position. Stop when top of mattress is level with elbows.
3. Palms up, slide one hand under the child's back and grasp his shoulder. Press forearms against mattress while sliding arm under child. Slide the other hand under his thighs and grasp his hip.
4. Use your arms as a sled. Shift weight to the rear leg and draw the child to the edges of the bed.

### Caution

A heavy person need not be moved all at once. It is easier to bring over the head and shoulders, the hips, and then the legs, one unit at a time.

Do not lift from this position.

### Additional Considerations

Follow the same steps when moving the child to the side of the therapy table. Hold a child who has a great deal of involuntary motion close to you when he is on the edge of the bed.

See if the bed can be raised with blocks to lessen the strain.

## LIFTING CHILD WITHOUT BRACES FROM BED

1. Start with the child at the edge of the bed.
2. Stand close to the bed with the knees bent.

3. Raise the child to a sitting position.
4. Place one arm around the child's back under his upper arm and grasp him over his forearm.
5. Place the other arm under his knees.
6. Gather the child to your chest and rise to a standing position by straightening your knees. Child should bend hips, knees, and neck as much as possible.

### Additional Considerations

If the child is light, simply squat and draw the child to your chest. Rise by straightening your legs.

If the bed is low, draw the child onto the thigh and lift him to your waist level. Consider raising the bed by using blocks.

## LIFTING CHILD WITH LONG BRACES FROM BED

1. Draw covers completely away from the child before starting lift.
2. Stand next to the bed with your legs spread and your hips and knees bent so that your elbows are near bed level.
3. Slide one hand under the child's chest, then under his upper arm and grasp him over his forearm.
4. With the other hand grasping under the thighs, draw the child next to your body.
5. Straighten hips and knees, keeping your elbows drawn back and your forearms upward toward your chest to hold the child close. Child should bend his hips, knees, and neck as much as possible.

### Additional Consideration

If the bed is extremely low, the child can be drawn against the thigh. Then the child is lifted to a carrying position, with a helping upward knee thrust for a heavy child.

## LIFTING HEAVY CHILD WITHOUT BRACES FROM FLOOR TO STANDING POSITION

1. Kneel close behind the child and grasp him under his armpits, with the grasp pressure against the trunk.
2. Raise the child to a sitting position.
3. Shift to a stride position with your knees bent and back straight.
4. Still grasping child under armpits, raise him to a standing position by straightening your legs and shifting your weight quickly toward your rear foot.

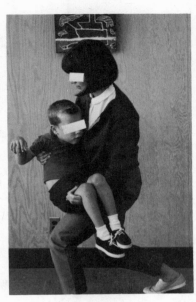

**FIG. 4-3.** Lifting child from floor. Most of child's weight rests on aide's thigh. Back is kept straight. (From Svirsky, H. S. The severely involved child: Maternal backache. *Clin Orthop 47*:58, 1966. Reproduced with permission)

In this way the child's back will slide up your supporting leg.
5. Give him crutches or a cane or transfer him to a wheelchair or a chair with wheels added if he cannot walk unsupported.

### Additional Considerations

If the child is lighter, crouch low at his side with knees bent. Grasping him beneath his shoulders and under his thighs, draw him close to your body and rise to a standing position by straightening your legs.

In picking up a lighter child from the floor, allow most of his weight to rest on your thigh. Raise him with arm-and-leg action while your spine remains straight (Fig. 4-3).

### LIFTING HEAVY CHILD WITH BRACES FROM FLOOR TO STANDING POSITION

1. Crouch near the child's head and place the hands under the child's back and shoulders to lift him to a sitting position.
2. Squat and grasp the child's braces at his hip.
3. Rise to a bent-knee position, maintaining firm grasp.

4. Draw the child's trunk onto your thigh by shifting your weight toward the rear.
5. Straighten your legs and shift weight over forward foot, drawing the child to a standing position with his weight resting on your thigh.
6. Stand close to the child and hold him in a balanced position.

### Additional Considerations

If the child is light, crouch at his side with knees bent. Grasping him beneath his shoulders and under his thighs, draw him close to your body and rise to a standing position by straightening your legs.

### LIFTING CHILD FROM WHEELCHAIR TO STANDING POSITION

1. Apply wheelchair brakes. Face the child.
2. Crouch to swing footrests into vertical position, out of the way of the child's feet.
3. Stand in a bent-knee position with forward leg between the child's knees, and place your hands about the child's waist or under his armpits.
4. Shift your weight backward over the rear foot as you slide the child to the front of the seat.
5. Have the child lean forward and keep his weight over his feet as you draw him up to a standing position. It may help if he holds your hips or shoulders.

### ASSISTING CHILD TO WALK DURING CHANGE OF POSITION

If the child is able to support his weight on his legs and is able to take steps but has difficulty in maintaining his balance, assist him as follows:
1. Stand close behind him so that your forward leg is in contact with the child.
2. Grasp his waist or the waistband of his brace with one hand. Place your other hand over his shoulder or under his armpit.
3. As the child moves forward, keep your hand and leg in contact with him.
4. Use your leg to assist the child in moving forward by swinging the leg forward against his buttock in a lifting motion (Fig. 4-4).

### ASSISTING CHILD WHO HAS LOST HIS BALANCE

If the child starts to fall while walking, step close to him and place your leg next to him for support or to break his fall. If at all possible, grasp his clothing or

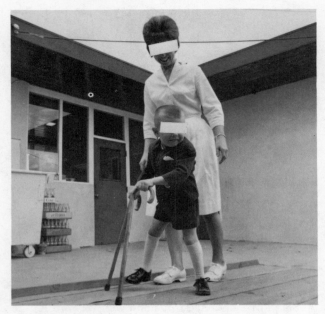

**FIG. 4-4.** Assisting child to walk. Attendant's right leg is pushing against child's buttock, giving support while helping him to move forward. (Courtesy UCP of Denver, 1966. Reproduced with permission)

trunk, and as his body is lowered, shift your weight away from the direction of his fall and draw him against your supporting leg.

If the child is falling toward you, crouch and place one leg under him or place your thigh against him while supporting his upper trunk with your hands.

### Caution

The goal should be to prevent injury, not to regain balance. Do not reach outward or lean over to catch him.

### ASSISTING CHILD TO WALK DOWNSTAIRS

1. At the top of the stairs, place the child's hand or both hands on the rail, and while steadying him, move to the step below him and face him.
2. Grasp the child's waist and move to the next lower step. Stay close to the railing. Keep your weight forward. Rest your arm and hip against the rail.
3. Guide the child as he moves to the step below him. Let him steady himself on each step.
4. Move to the next lower step and repeat the actions listed above.

### Caution

Keep your entire foot on the step if possible. If balance is lost, lean toward the railing and grasp it with one hand while holding the child with the other hand. Have him sit down and rest if he becomes over-excited during the descent.

### LIFTING WHEELCHAIR INTO AUTOMOBILE

1. Move car seat forward.
2. Collapse the wheelchair close to the car door and face it toward the opening behind the front seat.
3. Tilt the chair until the front wheels mount the floor of the car and the large wheels rest against the edge of the car.
4. Stand with the legs in a stride position with the knees bent.
5. Lift the wheelchair, using your legs, as the wheelchair is rolled on its front wheels onto the floor of the automobile.
6. Guide the wheelchair into the automobile by advancing the weight over the forward leg.

**FIG. 4-5.** Carrying child. The hips bear child's weight, and slight backward lean helps to counterbalance the weight. (From Svirsky, H. S. The severely involved child: Maternal backache. *Clin Orthop 47:*58, 1966. Reproduced with permission)

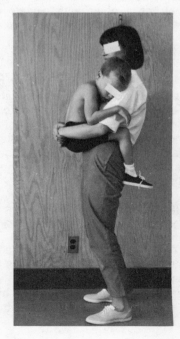

## Additional Considerations

If the wheelchair's drive wheels are forward, turn the chair so that the handles are toward the automobile and the drive wheels are against the side of the automobile. Enter the automobile and, with the legs in a stride position, crouch and grasp the handles of the wheelchair. Draw the wheelchair into the automobile by shifting the weight to the rear.

## REMOVING WHEELCHAIR FROM AUTOMOBILE

In a one-door car, push the front seat forward.
1. Align rear of wheelchair with opening behind the front seat and move it close to the edge of the automobile.
2. From outside the car, stand with the legs in a stride position.
3. Grasp the handles and tilt the chair backward.
4. Draw the chair to the edge of the car by shifting the weight to the rear leg. Roll the chair on its large wheels.
5. Crouch and control the descent of the chair by forcing the wheels against the edge of the car as the chair is lowered.

## LIFTING WHEELCHAIR INTO AUTO TRUNK

1. Open car trunk and collapse the wheelchair.
2. Stand in a stride position at right angles to the chair with your feet facing toward car trunk.
3. Bend the knees and tilt the folded chair against the thighs.
   frame, not by any movable part such as wheel or
4. Take a low grasp on the chair. Grasp chair by frame, not by any movable part such as wheel or arms. In a continuous motion straighten your legs and place the chair into the car trunk.
5. Stand close to the automobile and slide the chair into the trunk.

## Alternative Method

Sometimes it is easier to lift the chair onto a low box. Lean the chair against the trunk, lift lower end to a horizontal position and slide it into the trunk. This may take longer, but it preserves your back. Bend knees to take a low grasp.

## REMOVING WHEELCHAIR FROM AUTO TRUNK

1. Stand close and grasp chair frame.

2. Slide wheelchair outward by shifting your weight to the rear.
3. Tilt chair to an upright position and roll it backward over the rear of the auto trunk.
4. Lower chair to the ground by sliding it along your thigh as the knees bend until it rests on the ground.

## CARRYING

### PRINCIPLES OF GOOD CARRYING

1. Avoid carrying whenever possible by using a household chair with wheels added, tricycles, wheelchairs, or hydraulic lifts.
2. When carrying is absolutely necessary, hold the load as close to your chest as possible.
3. Keep a firm grasp. If your grasp becomes loose, rest the child against something while you secure a firmer grasp.
4. Keep your back straight, not arched—either forward or backward.
5. Do not twist; turn your whole body.

### CARRYING A CHILD WITHOUT TIGHT ADDUCTORS

1. Keep your arms close to your body.
2. Rest part of child's weight on your hips and counterbalance his weight by leaning back from slightly flexed knees, without hypertension of lumbar spine (Fig. 4-5).
3. Have child lean against you, since he cannot help by holding your shoulders.

### CARRYING A CHILD HORIZONTALLY, IF NECESSARY

1. Hold the child with one of your arms under his knees and the other under his chest, your palms facing upward.
2. Hold the child tightly against your body to relieve arm strain and prevent shifting.
3. Take short steps to maintain balance; do not walk fast.
4. Keep your hips under the load of your upper body and the child.
5. Walk with a large share of the weight over your heels.
6. To carry a heavy child for short distances, support his weight against your upper thighs. Keep your hips slightly flexed.

## CARRYING LARGE CHILD VERTICALLY

1. Place the child on a step or firm step stool. If possible, have him step up himself while supported.
2. Clasp your hands under child's buttocks, holding his arms down with yours (Fig. 4-6).
3. Have him lean against you with his head over one of your shoulders.
4. Hold him close, with his weight well over your heels.
5. Going up bus step, shift your weight well over your front. Coming down bus step, rest the child's weight against the bus door while descending. Keep weight over leg supporting child and bend supporting knee as other leg makes the step downward. A firm grasp prevents child's weight from shifting during this process.

## CARRYING CHILD UPSTAIRS

1. Walk close to the railing and rest against it if support is needed.
2. Bend forward at your hips, to use the strong hip muscles.
3. Place your entire foot on each stair tread, *not* just the front tip.
4. Child should assist, if possible, by holding onto your neck and shoulder.

## CARRYING CHILD DOWNSTAIRS

1. Stay close to the handrail and rest against it for support.
2. Bend knees slightly to keep balance.
3. Place the entire foot on each stair tread. Keep weight back.
4. If a handrail is against the wall, the wall can be used also to rest against and to help keep balance.
5. Do not hurry.
6. Child should assist, if able, by placing his arm around your neck.

## TWO PEOPLE CARRYING CHILD

Two people can carry one child easily by supporting the child between them.
1. The carriers stand on either side of the child, both facing the same direction. Each carrier encircles the child's waist with the arm nearest the child and grasps under one of the child's thighs with one hand.
2. Stand close.

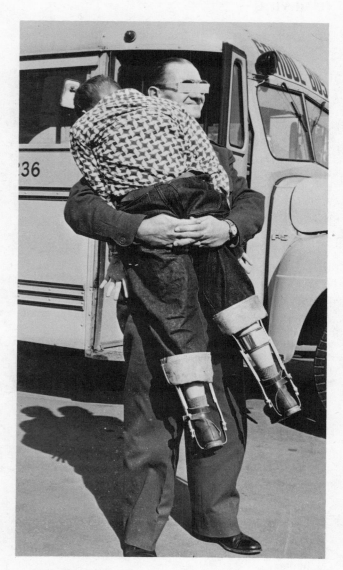

**FIG. 4-6.** Carrying large child in vertical position. Aide's arms are clasped firmly under child's buttocks, holding down his arms. (From Assisting the Cerebral Palsied Child: Lifting and Carrying)

3. Distribute weight evenly by holding the child upright in a sitting position.
4. Take short steps, in rhythm if possible.
5. Child should assist, if able, by placing his arms over the carriers' shoulders.

### Additional Considerations

A child with a great deal of involuntary motion should be carried with his arms pressed against carriers' waists.

If the child is in braces, the carriers may find it easier to grasp the brace at the child's thigh and at his back.

## SHIFTING HORIZONTALLY CARRIED CHILD FROM ONE ARM TO THE OTHER

1. Cradle child firmly about his shoulders with one hand. Shift your weight slightly to your foot on the same side while you step backward on it.
2. Draw child's chest close and lower his legs with your opposite arm.
3. Transfer your arm that is under his legs to an overarm grasp while crouching to rest the child's weight against your thigh.
4. Lower the child's legs and shift him to a vertical position, and at the same time transfer your hand that is holding the legs to a position below the child's buttocks.
5. Support the child with your hand that is beneath his buttocks and shift the child's head to your opposite shoulder.
6. Move your upper hand to grasp the child's thighs and move your hand beneath his buttocks upward to his waist.
7. Shift your weight to your leg in back position and raise the child to a higher carrying position.
8. Shift your arm holding the child's thighs until it goes under them, palm up. His head is now resting on your opposite shoulder (Fig. 4-7).

## FALLING WHILE CARRYING

1. If close to a wall or other stable object, rest weight on it.
2. Be alert to protect the child's head.
3. Fall under or to the side of child.
4. Turn child away from hard objects.
5. Fall against the bed or other soft object if close.
6. If falling downstairs, try to lower to sitting position on step.

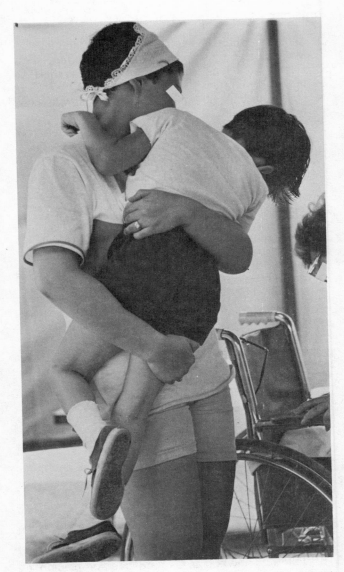

**FIG. 4-7.** Shifting child from one arm to the other. Hand that was in upper position has been moved to his thighs, while lower hand was moved up to the child's waist. (Courtesy of United Cerebral Palsy Association of Nassau County, Roosevelt, N.Y.)

7. If falling upstairs, turn and sit on the stairs, holding onto the child.
8. After stumbling, crouch and sit down to prevent tumbling.

## LOWERING

### PRINCIPLES OF GOOD LOWERING

1. Make sure there is ample room for good footing.
2. Make sure your grasp is firm before lowering.
3. Spread your legs to hip width and lower the load between your feet.
4. Hold your back straight and steady, even when you lean far forward.
5. Lower in a slow and even manner by bending your legs.
6. Extend your arms straight downward and keep the load close to your body.
7. Do not twist your body. To turn, move your feet.

### LOWERING CHILD TO BED

1. Stand a few inches from the bed with legs apart.
2. Lower the child, holding him against your body, and bend your forward knee until it rests against the bed.
3. Slide the child down your thighs and onto the bed.
4. Adjust the child in the bed from a bent-knee position.

### LOWERING CHILD TO CHAIR

1. Stand close to the side of the chair.
2. Lower to a bent-knee position and keep your trunk erect.
3. Extend your arms and slide the child down your thigh onto the seat of the chair. Avoid twisting while lowering the child.
4. Squat and adjust the child's position in the chair.

### PLACING CHILD IN WHEELCHAIR

Stabilize the wheelchair before bringing child to it. Apply brakes; place the back of the wheelchair against the wall or other stable object or block the wheels. The following method is a good one for placing a medium-sized child into a wheelchair if the adult has strong arms, shoulders, and trunk. The trunk is kept straight and not twisted, and some weight is transmitted to the left hip.

1. Carry the child to the front of the wheelchair.
2. Lower the child to a standing position close to the wheelchair.
3. Standing close to the corner of the wheelchair in a bent-knee position, seat the child in the wheelchair (Fig. 4-8).

**Alternative Method**

A weaker adult might stand close in front of the child, whose back is to the wheelchair, flex her knees, straddling the child, and pick him up by extending her knees.

### LOWERING CHILD TO TOILET

The toilet seat should be kept down and the lid up.
1. With child in your arms, stand close and slightly to one side of toilet.
2. Step forward on leg farthest from toilet and lower yourself to a bent-knee position. Lower the child's feet to the floor and rest his chest against your thigh.
3. Squat and encircle the child's body with one arm while the other hand is used to adjust the child's clothing.
4. Maintaining a grasp on the child, rise to a bent-knee position. Keep your back straight.
5. With one arm, encircle the child's waist and grasp under his thigh with your other hand. Straighten your legs and place the child onto the toilet seat.
6. Crouch and adjust child's position.

### REMOVING CHILD FROM TOILET

1. Take a bent-knee stride position close to the toilet.
2. Encircle the child's waist with one arm and grasp his thigh with your opposite hand. Draw child off seat by shifting your weight to your foot at the rear.
3. Squat and rest the child against your shoulder while adjusting his clothes.
4. Lift child to carrying position.

### LOWERING CHILD TO BATHTUB

If possible, use a chair in a shower stall, rather than a bathtub. Delay filling the tub until the child is in it. Drape a damp towel over the side of the tub. Fold a bath mat to provide a knee pad on the floor below the towel. Place a heavy rubber mat with suction in the tub.
1. Lower the child's legs into the tub and seat the

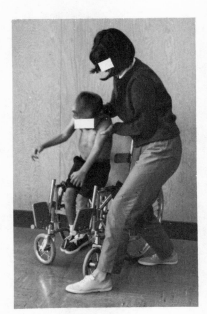

**FIG. 4-8.** Placing child in wheelchair. Aide is in a stride position, knees bent, close to corner of chair, so that as child is lifted into chair, her weight may be shifted. (From Svirsky, H. W. The severely involved child: Maternal backache. *Clin Orthop 47:*59, 1966. Reproduced with permission)

child on the towel on the side of the tub. This is accomplished by bending your knees and allowing the child to slide feet first down your thigh onto the tub.
2. Rise and shift your grasp to underneath the child's shoulders.
3. Lower to a squatting position while holding the child's back against the side of the tub as the child and the towel slide into the tub.
4. Kneel on the mat while arranging the child's position and bathing him.

### Additional Considerations

If the child can grasp, put bars on the wall or tub side.

Where possible, lean against the wall while lowering the child, to relieve some of the weight.

If the child is heavy secure the assistance of another person. A very heavy child should be given sponge baths if no assistance can be obtained.

If the child can sit by himself, an aluminum or wood chair can be placed in the tub and the child washed using a hose and spray.

## REMOVING CHILD FROM BATHTUB

Drain the tub, then dry the child. Drape the damp towel over the side of the tub.
1. In a crouch position, place the child's back against the towel, using an underarm grasp.
2. Shifting the weight to the rear, slide the child up the side of the tub onto your thigh.
3. Holding the child close with one hand, slide the other hand under his legs and draw him toward your chest in a carrying position.

### Additional Considerations

If the child is light, he may be raised from the tub in a carrying position. First, bring him to the edge of the tub and rest him there.

A heavy child is best held under his chest and under his legs; push him against towel at side of tub and slide him up and over the edge of the tub.

Sometimes it is easier to stand in the tub to lift the child, but if the child is heavy enough to make this necessary, consider showering him on a tub seat or giving him a sponge bath.

## REFERENCES

Svirsky, H. S. "The severely involved child: Maternal backache," *Clin Orthop* 47:57–64, 1966.

Cooper, J., Morehouse, L. E. "Assisting the Cerebral Palsied Child: Lifting and Carrying," United Cerebral Palsy Association, Inc. 1953. (out of print)

Cicenia, E. F., Hoberman, M., Dervits, H. L. "Safety: A factor in Functional Training of the Disabled Child," *Phys Ther Rev* 40:5: 337–368, 1960.

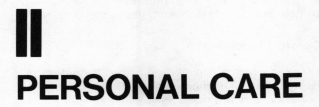

# PERSONAL CARE

# 5
# Feeding and Eating Equipment

Feeding and eating are not ends in themselves. They are a means toward good nutrition and toward exercising the muscles that will eventually be used in speech. They also provide one of the pleasurable activities of mankind. Therefore, several aids in feeding and eating for patients with cerebral palsy will be discussed in this chapter. It must be remembered, however, that they are only *aids* and that other factors are important. A list of professional guides is included in the References for additional information.

**General Precautions**

1. Guard against aspiration of food. Do not allow a child to lie flat when drinking. Do not tip his head back and pour liquids down while he is in a reclining position. Do not allow child to swallow when he is in extensor thrust position instead of a flexed position or seated tailor-fashion to counteract opisthotonos (arched extended back position).
2. Do not allow a child to swallow chunks of undigestible food. Ask the doctor or nurse to give you a list of solids, such as bananas and skinless frank-

furters, that are more digestible if they are accidentally swallowed in chunks.

3. Do not make feeding a tug of war between two personalities, rather than a pleasurable time. Consider feeding in small frequent sessions, rather than three main meals; giving a child a variety of plates containing small bites to be taken in his fingers; giving supplemented milk (add powdered milk or nutrient, such as Carnation Breakfast).

4. Do not feed a child in order to "save time" if he can eat certain foods himself when he is properly positioned and given ample time. Provide enough space for him to get a little messy while eating.

## SUCKING AIDS FOR SUPINE FEEDING

Whether the child is in a supine position or sitting up, a variety of aids to feeding, are available or may be devised to encourage sucking.

### PLASTIC BOTTLE WITH NIPPLE

A plastic wide-neck nursing bottle may be fitted with several types of nipples and aids that help an infant learn to close his lips successfully. The child can then progressively learn to suck on a plastic straw. The nipple should be sufficiently firm to encourage sucking. The holes in the nipple should be small so that the liquid does not flow into the child by mere gravity. A gentle squeeze on the plastic bottle (Fig. 5-1) will give positive reinforcement to the child's attempts to suck, preventing frustration.

### NUK SAUGER NIPPLE

Use this nipple (Fig. 5-2) with the Nuk Sauger bottle or other wide-mouthed bottles. If the child has poor lip closure, a slight pressure causes the soft bulbar flare to press against the lips. This prevents air leakage and helps create a vacuum that draws liquid up.

### Precautions

1. Do not enlarge the nipple hole.
2. Use cold sterilization since the nipple softens with boiling.
3. For infants with poor sucking ability, use a plastic bottle with the Nuk Sauger nipple. Slight pressure on the bottle will help the child's sucking attempt by producing a fine, controlled stream of formula.

### Source

Rocky Mountain Dental Products Co.

### DAVOL WING NIPPLE

This nipple fits the Even-Flo bottle and is held securely by nipple holders which fasten over the flange (Fig. 5-3). It is available at any drugstore.

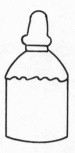

**FIG. 5-1.** A plastic bottle with nipple. A firm nipple with small holes will encourage sucking. (Courtesy of U. Haynes, United Cerebral Palsy Associations, Inc., New York)

**FIG. 5-2.** A Nuk-Sauger nipple, with bulbar flare to prevent air leakage. (Courtesy of U. Haynes, United Cerebral Palsy Associations, Inc., New York)

**FIG. 5-3.** A Davol Wing nipple, showing flange holder. (Courtesy of U. Haynes, United Cerebral Palsy Associations, Inc., New York)

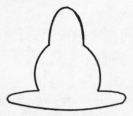

**FIG. 5-4.** Standard bottle nipple. Several adaptations make this a suitable sucking aid. (Courtesy of U. Haynes, United Cerebral Palsy Associations, Inc., New York)

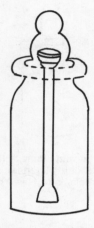

**FIG. 5-5.** Standard nipple used with Sit-Up plastic straw insert especially designed for sucking in upright position. (Courtesy of U. Haynes, United Cerebral Palsy Associations, Inc., New York)

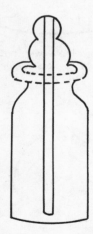

**FIG. 5-6.** Standard nipple with hole made to hold plastic straw firmly. (Courtesy of U. Haynes, United Cerebral Palsy Associations, Inc., New York)

## SUCKING AIDS FOR SITTING-UP FEEDING

The standard nipple (Fig. 5-4) may be fitted with sucking aids. These are often called "heads-up" sucking aids to describe the child's position when sucking. The child can be taught to suck and swallow while sitting with his head upright or flexed slightly forward. Try the "nipple straw" inserts before purchasing other equipment. Practice snug fit between the top of the nipple straw and the nipple to avoid air leakage at their juncture. Most Curity nipples fit well.

### STANDARD NIPPLE WITH SIT-UP OR SIT-N-SIP

This insert (Fig. 5-5) fits best in Curity nipples and fits standard wide-neck bottles, like Even-Flo and Curity. Plastic bottles permit slight positive pressure, when indicated, to reward sucking attempts with a gentle flow of liquid. Keep nipple holes small to encourage true sucking motions. Use nonbrittle plastic straws.

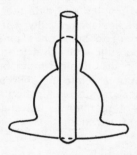

**FIG. 5-7.** Straw protruding through nipples to encourage use of straw rather than nipple. (Courtesy of U. Haynes, United Cerebral Palsy Associations, Inc., New York)

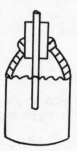

**FIG. 5-8.** Straw held tightly by bottle stopper to encourage use of straw. (Courtesy of U. Haynes, United Cerebral Palsy Associations, Inc., New York)

## Sources

Medi, Inc. (Sit-N-Sip)
Noair Manufacturing Co. (Sit Up)

## STANDARD NIPPLE WITH PLASTIC STRAW INSERT

After using the devices mentioned above, the child may progress slowly to the use of a plastic straw inserted into a nipple. The straw must reach from the bottom of the bottle up into the sucking part of the nipple. A hole must be made in the nipple to hold the straw firmly (Fig. 5-6). The nipple of the Infa-Feeder may also be used to hold the straw.

Slight pressure on the plastic bottle, at first, helps the liquid rise when lip closure and sucking are still weak. Gentle stimulation around the lips or gently helping lips to close around the straw may also prove helpful in early training.

The straw may be made to protrude from the bottle, just a bit at first (Fig. 5-7), and then the projection slowly increased until the child is sucking entirely through the straw.

The plastic straws (nonbrittle, with wide or narrow holes) can be found in most drugstores and supermarkets.

## BOTTLE WITH STRAW

The bottle with a straw (Fig. 5-8) is useful when the child changes from the nipple or the nipple with straw insert. The straw is inserted through a rubber stopper.

### Precautions

1. Stopper must fit the bottle snugly.
2. Hole in the stopper must be a tight fit for the straw to prevent air leakage that could make sucking difficult.
3. Use a nonbrittle type of plastic straw. It has a soft touch to the lips.

### Construction

1. A small plastic nursing bottle is best. Less energy is required to draw liquid up a short straw in a small bottle.
2. A rubber stopper, of a diameter to fit the bottle neck, is inserted into the bottle and tested for snug fit. Stopper must have a hole in the center for the straw. Be careful not to have too large a hole.

3. A plastic straw, 4 to 5 inches long, is inserted through the hole in the stopper. The fit must be tight.

## INFA-FEEDER

For infants with a strong backward thrust, the Infa-Feeder is useful (Fig. 5-9). It can also be used as an intermediate step between bottle and spoon feeding. Thicker foods can be used in the Infa-Feeder than in the bottle. It has a plunger that is used to force the bottle contents into the nipple. The child should be in a side-lying position with a small pillow under the head. As the child relaxes, bring the head from backward thrust into line with the body. Use strained foods prescribed for him, and push plunger gently upward to refill the nipple as he swallows. His attempts to suck again will thus be rewarded.

### Precautions

1. Do not use plunger to push food into the child's mouth. Place him in a position to suck food out of the nipple.
2. Prevent any chance of his breathing food or liquid into the windpipe by controlling arched back and backward thrust of the head.
3. Do not rush. Give the child time to suck food out of the nipple before refilling the nipple.

### Source

Deemer-Howard Associates, Inc.

**FIG. 5-9.** Infa-Feeder, in which thicker foods can be given than in a bottle. (Courtesy of U. Haynes, United Cerebral Palsy Associations, Inc., New York)

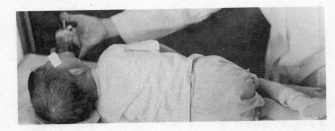

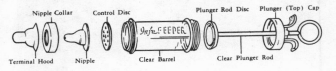

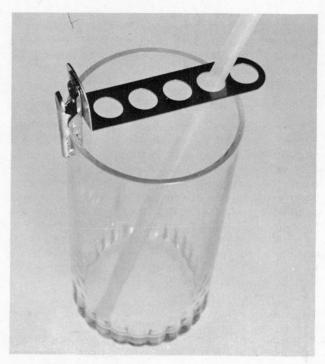

FIG. 5-10. Stainless steel holder clipped onto glass to hold drinking straw in place. (Courtesy of Fred Sammons, Inc., Brookfield, Ill.)

FIG. 5-11. Proper position of child for lap feeding. (Courtesy of U. Haynes, United Cerebral Palsy Associations, Inc., New York)

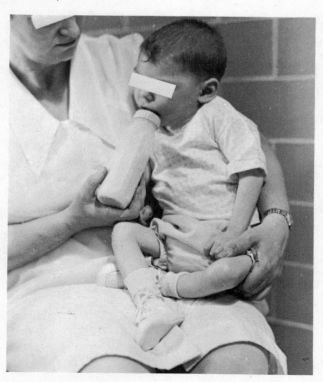

# STRAW HOLDERS

There are several devices available to hold drinking straws in place on a cup or glass, or a holder can be made. Such an aid is a necessity for the young child or for the person unable to use or to control his hands.

## DRINKING STRAW HOLDER B-K 1126

This stainless steel holder clamps conveniently on the lip of any glass (Fig. 5-10). Large drinking straws will not fit, however.

**Source**

Fred Sammons, Inc.

## PLASTIC CONTAINER WITH COVER

A plastic container of 4-ounce size is desirable with a lid. It is firm but will yield to slight pressure without dislocating the cover.

## PLASTIC REFRIGERATOR CUP WITH LID

A small plastic refrigerator cup with a lid into which a hole is made to accommodate a straw is useful. The 4½-ounce size with a lid of Falcon Plastics is firm but has enough "give" to yield to gentle pressure and aid sucking.

## PLASTIC SQUEEZE BOTTLE WITH PLASTIC STRAW

Plastic squeeze bottles may be obtained in any variety store or pharmacy. Get plastic tubing 3/16 inch in diameter. Many tropical fish stores and hardware stores sell such tubing. Cut an opening in the top of the squeeze bottle the exact diameter of the tubing and insert a strip of the tubing for a plastic straw.

## BULL DOG CLIP STRAW HOLDER

Clip a large paper clip to the side of a glass. Bend the finger section of the clip that is on the inside of the glass toward a 90-degree angle from the other finger section. Place plastic tubing through the loop created by this bend, using a piece long enough to reach the bottom of the glass and the patient's mouth when the glass is held at a convenient drinking position.

## PENCIL CLIP STRAW HOLDER

A standard pocket pencil clip, available at any stationery store, can be clipped to the side of the glass. Pass the straw through the section of the clip that usually holds the pencil.

## PROPER POSITIONING FOR LAP FEEDING

Proper positioning for lap feeding controls extensor thrust and prevents the child's head from falling backward (Fig. 5-11). One arm of the child is held against the adult while the adult holds the other arm close to the child's body. The child sits tailor-fashion on the lap.

## ADAPTED EATING UTENSILS

Only through trial and error can one select the best utensil for a given child (Fig. 5-12). Commercial items are of two types: utensils made with bulky handles, or holders that cling to the user's hand and hold the utensil slipped into them.

## BUILT-UP HANDLE UTENSILS

These nonswiveling utensils are light weight, with large plastic handles (Fig. 5-13).

### Source

J. A. Preston Corp.

## EXPANDLE UTENSILS

A feather-weight aluminum handle attached to the utensil can be easily bent to the size and shape needed for the individual patient (Fig. 5-14). The utensils are stainless steel.

### Source

Fred Sammons, Inc.

## UTENSIL HOLDER

This holder, which comes in three models, is basically a band which fastens around the user's palm to substitute for grasp (Fig. 5-15). The utensil slips into a pouch on the band.

**FIG. 5-12.** Eating utensils from which suitable instrument should be selected. (*1*) Wooden dowel with plastic-covered spoon inserted. (*2*) Curved baby spoon. (*3*) Curved stainless steel teaspoon. (*4*) Dee-Scoop spoon, available for right or left hand. (*5*) Left-handed Dee-Scoop spoon. (*6*) Plastic baby spoon, curved. (*7*) Stainless steel ladle with spout. (*8*) Child's spoon with plastic handle. (*9*) Plastic fork with wrist strap. (*10*) Curved fork with large handle. (*11*) Wide fork with plastic handle. (*12*) Plastic teaspoon. (*13*) Fork with large handle. (*14*) Ordinary fork, curved. (From Bensberg, G. J., ed. *Teaching the Mentally Retarded: A Handbook for Ward Personnel.* Atlanta, Southern Regional Education Board, 1966. Reprinted with permission)

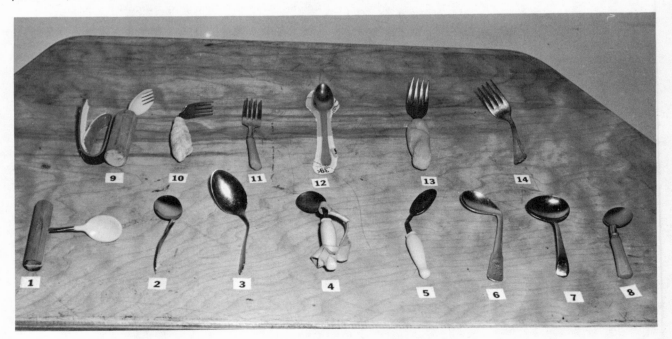

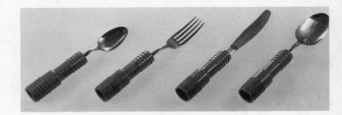

**FIG. 5-13.** Built-up handle utensils. Ridges in the plastic are an aid to grasping. (Copyright 1965 by J. A. Preston Corporation)

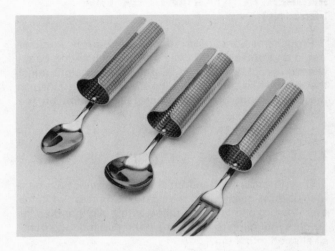

**FIG. 5-14.** Expandle utensils. Light-weight aluminum handles are easily bent to required shape. (Courtesy of Fred Sammons, Inc., Brookfield, Ill.)

**FIG. 5-15.** Utensil holders for palm of hand. All have Velcro closures. Model 1050, all plastic; Model 1052, plastic with elastic insert for better fit; Models 1053, 1054, and 1055, economy models in various sizes, with strong elastic bands. (Courtesy of Fred Sammons, Inc., Brookfield, Ill.)

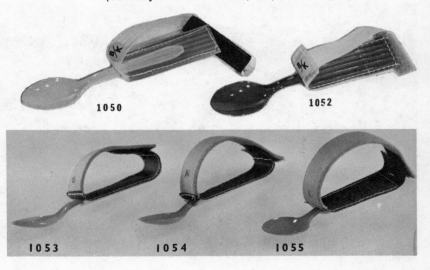

**Source**

Fred Sammons, Inc.

## HOME-MADE UTENSIL HOLDING AIDS

Bulky handles make eating utensils easier to grasp. Bulk without too much weight can be added by inserting handle into a large empty spool, pushing it through a foam rubber ball, attaching sponge or plastic foam, or taping foam rubber strips around the handle (Fig. 5-16). Grasp can also be improved by bending the handle of the utensil or attaching Velcro and then winding it around the palm.

One convenient way of adding bulk is to build up the handle with Aircast. This material looks like bandage. It is soluble in acetone and then hardens. Within 24 hours it can withstand high temperatures so that the utensil can be placed in a dishwasher or sterilizer. One small roll of Aircast makes 10 or 12 built-up handles on spoons.

**Source of Material**

The Tower Company, Inc.

## UTENSILS THAT WILL MINIMIZE BRUISING

When the child bites down on a hard utensil, he may bruise his lips or gums. Ideas to prevent this follow.
1. Broad butter knife, rounded blade. This is good for solid food that will stay in a lump on the knife. The child can bite down without hurting himself.
2. Plastic fork. Plastic picnic fork may be inserted into a bite-size piece of food; the child can manage alone from then on.
3. Spoon with Teflon or rubber coating. The coating smooths sharp edges. The spoon is available in supermarkets and in five-and-ten-cent stores.
4. Flexible rubber spoon. The soft, pliable rubber of this commercially available spoon will hold its shape even when boiled.

**Source**

Cleo Living Aids

## SANDWICH HOLDER

A sandwich holder (Fig. 5-17) eliminates crushing, dropping, or throwing the sandwich. It can hold a quarter of a sandwich or a piece of meat.

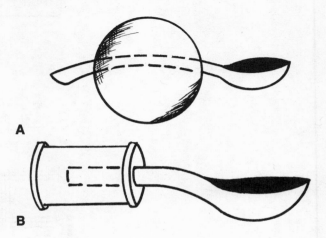

**FIG. 5-16.** Home-made bulky handles for spoons. (*A*) Ball, (*B*) Spool.

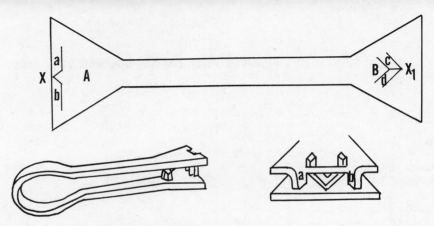

**FIG. 5-17.** Diagram for construction of sandwich holder. *Top,* points cut at *X* and *X₁;* teeth, *a, b, c, d;* surface of holder *A* and *B. Bottom left,* side view, and *right,* front view, showing how teeth will hold food. (Courtesy New York University Medical Center of the Institute of Rehabilitation Medicine)

**FIG. 5-18.** Diagram for long-handled holder. *Top,* side view; *center,* top view; *bottom left,* end view; *bottom right,* detail of hinge. See text for explanation. (Courtesy of the New York University Medical Center Institute for Rehabilitation Medicine)

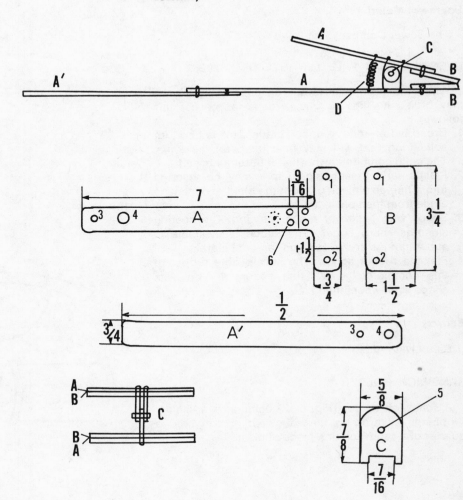

## Construction

1. Cut a strip of aluminum and carefully file edges smooth.
2. Cut at points X and X₁ to free teeth *a, b, c,* and *d.*
3. Bend teeth perpendicularly to surfaces *A* and *B.*
4. Bend strip so that teeth can meet and lock, holding food in place.

## LONG-HANDLED HOLDER

Another holder that can be constructed (Fig. 5-18) is intended primarily to hold a sandwich or a wash-cloth, but it can be used also for a handkerchief, powder puff, or any object desired near the face by the patient unable to raise his arms. It is made of aluminum with plastic end pieces for sanitary grip, and has a steel spring for tight gripping action. The handle can be extended once or twice its own length and is held firm by a dimple lock.

## Construction

*A*, handles. Cut two pieces, one 3 inches shorter; use ⅟₁₆-inch st aluminum.

*A'*, handle extension. Cut one piece from ⅟₁₆-inch 24 st aluminum.

*B*, end plates. Cut two pieces from ⅛-inch Plexiglas.

*C*, hinge. Cut three pieces·from ³⁄₃₂-inch aluminum.

*D*, compression spring. Made from 0.041 piano wire, wound on ³⁄₁₆-inch mandrel with ³⁄₃₂-inch spacing of turns.

*1, 2, 3*, rivets, ⅛-inch diameter aluminum.

*4*, dimple lock. Convex surface made by insertion of rivet; concave surface made by compressing a dent in surface of metal.

*1, 2, 3, 4*, holes (Fig. 5-19, *center, A*) are ⅛-inch diameter for rivets and dimple lock. Holes *3* and *4* are ¾ inch apart on both *A* and *A'*.

*5*, rivet in the detail showing part *C* is ³⁄₃₂-diameter aluminum and has a corresponding size hole, drilled ⁵⁄₁₆ inch below the top of the arch of part *C*.

*6*, rivets, ⁷⁄₁₆-inch diameter aluminum are drilled as shown, on the two pieces of part *A*.

## ADAPTED CUPS AND GLASSES

### General Precautions

1. Do not use mouthpiece of cup to pour liquids down a child's throat.
2. Encourage the child to sip from the cup.

## SPILL-PROOF DRINKING CUP

Made of shatter-proof plastic, this cup comes with two training lids to avoid spilling (Fig. 5-19). One has a slotted "see-through" lid; the other a "spout" style lid. There is a weighted base to keep the cup upright.

### Source

J. A. Preston Corp.

## ADJUSTABLE GLASS HOLDER

A holder that fits any size drinking glass (Fig. 5-20) has rubber grippers inside an adjustable stainless steel ring to assure a firm grip. The pliable plastic-coated handle may be bent to any hand size.

### Source

J. A. Preston Corp.

## SIPPIT

The Sippit, available in most drugstores, is an un-breakable plastic cup with a built-in short straw. It can be used as is, or a long straw can be inserted if the child has difficulty using the short mouthpiece.

## PLASTIC DRINKING MUG

This commercial drinking cup has a fine handle for persons with grasping problems (Fig. 5-21). It is of strong, durable plastic construction and comes in at-tractive assorted colors.

### Source

Fred Sammons, Inc.

## ADAPTED PLATES

Several types of plates are available, some made especially for the handicapped individual and some that can be used for the purpose, with or without special adaptations.

## CHILD'S HOT PLATE

A hot-water compartment to keep food warm is a feature of this shatter-proof plastic plate (Fig. 5-22). It has a suction cup base to hold it in place.

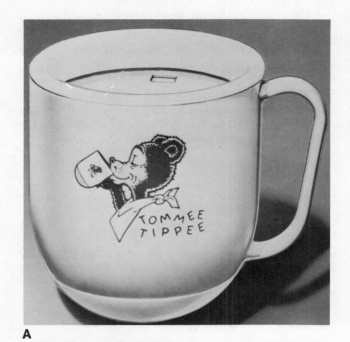

**A**

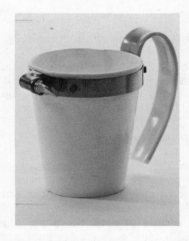

**FIG. 5-20.** Adjustable glass holder, for any size glass, with pliable handle. (Copyright 1965 by J. A. Preston Corporation)

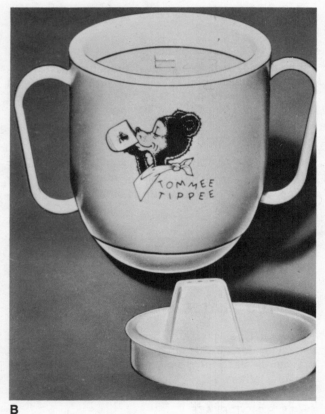

**B**

**FIG. 5-19.** Spill-proof Drinking Cup, with lid and weighted base, single handle (*A*) and twin handle (*B*). (Copyright 1965 by J. A. Preston Corporation)

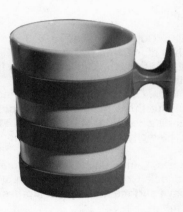

**FIG. 5-21.** Plastic drinking mug, with easily grasped handle. (Courtesy of Fred Sammons, Inc., Brookfield, Ill.)

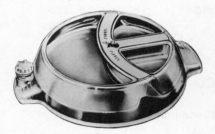

**FIG. 5-22.** A child's hot plate, with suction cup base. (Copyright 1965 by J. A. Preston Corporation)

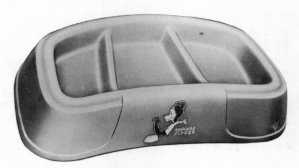

**FIG. 5-23.** Divided dish for child. (Copyright 1965 by J. A. Preston Corporation)

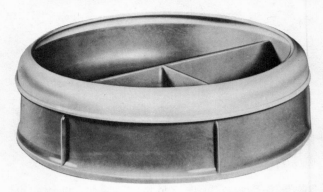

**FIG. 5-24.** Divided dish with guard rail to prevent spooning food overboard. (Copyright 1965 by J. A. Preston Corporation)

**FIG. 5-25.** Attachable food guards. *Top row: left,* No. 1090, clamps on back of plate; *center,* No. 1098, held by spring action; *right,* No. 1107 (old No. 1987), held by rubber bands and nonskid attachment. *Bottom row, left,* No. 1105, larger size held by spring action; *right,* No. 1112, Lazy Susan type. (Courtesy of Fred Sammons, Inc., Brookfield, Ill.)

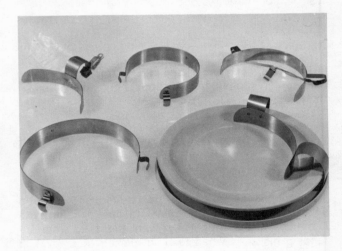

## Source

J. A. Preston Corp.

## BABY'S DIVIDED DISH

Two suction cups hold this dish firmly on the table or highchair tray (Fig. 5-23). It is made of shatterproof plastic and comes with baby's fork and spoon set made of plastic.

## Source

J. A. Preston Corp.

## DIVIDED DISH WITH GUARD RAIL

An instantly removable curved guard rail on this dish (Fig. 5-24) prevents food from being spooned overboard. Three suction cups hold the plastic dish on the table. It can also be used for adult patients.

## Source

J. A. Preston Corp.

## FOOD GUARDS

Several types of food guards are available (Fig. 5-25). Their main difference is in the mode of attachment. The Lazy Susan guard allows the plate to turn while the guard remains in place. The guards are made of stainless steel, electrically spot welded for durability.

## Source

Fred Sammons, Inc.

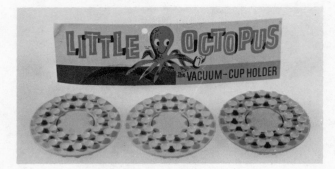

**FIG. 5-26.** Suction holders to hold dishes, glasses, etc. (Courtesy of Fred Sammons, Inc., Brookfield, Ill.)

## LITTLE OCTOPUS SUCTION HOLDER

The 30 tiny suction cups on each side of a soft rubber base provide a double-acting grip to anchor dishes, glasses, bowls, and many other items (Fig. 5-26). The holder is 3 inches in diameter by ⅜ inch thick. The tiny multiple suction cups replace larger, less reliable varieties of suction to hold table ware in place.

### Source

Fred Sammons, Inc. (The Little Octopus may also be available in kitchen gadget shops, hardware stores, or supermarkets.)

## SELF-FEEDING AIDS FOR CHILDREN

### ARM EXTENSION SUPPORT

Wooden book ends may be padded and covered with washable material. Fastened into position with C clamps, these supports prevent the child from extending his arms when feeding himself (Fig. 5-27). If arm abduction accompanies arm extension, an additional side may be added. The position of the supports can be varied to fit the individual user's needs.

### DISH STABILIZERS

Dishes can be held in place on the table or tray by several means:
1. A rubber mat can be placed under a dish.
2. A damp turkish towel, hand size or kitchen size, or a large washcloth can be tucked around a plate.

3. A circle of clay on a rubber-backed plastic mat will hold a plate that is firmly pressed down on it. Plasteline clay will stay soft longer.
4. The Little Octopus suction holder described above works very well.
5. Boards, with openings cut out to fit the bottoms of plates and cups, can be fastened to the table or tray with Little Octopus (see also Figure 5-29).

## TYPEWRITER PAD AS DISH STABILIZER

A typewriter pad with a nonskid base can also be used to hold plates in place. One that has proved useful is the Magic-Grip pad.

### Source

W. T. Rogers Co.

## BAKING PAN ADAPTATION FOR SCHOOL LUNCH USE

A square aluminum baking pan makes a highly satisfactory dish, especially for school lunch use (Fig. 5-28). Its straight sides make it easy for the child to

**FIG. 5-27.** Padded wooden book ends clamped to cut-out table to provide arm extension support. (Courtesy of P. Holser Buehler, United Cerebral Palsy Association of Los Angeles County)

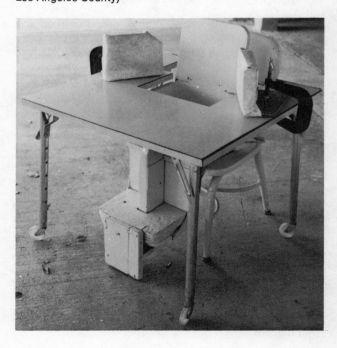

push food onto his spoon or fork. Moreover, it is easily cleaned by hand or in a dishwasher, and can stand up to the hard use in a lunchroom.

The pan is clamped to a wood board as a base. Hook clamps are fastened to the board with screws with wing nuts. The board itself is fastened to the table or desk with "C" clamps.

(The child using the dish in Figure 5-28 is holding a spoon with the handle enlarged with a wood dowel; the spoon has been bent to the child's requirement.)

Other useful adaptations may be made in this equipment, depending on the needs.

1. The user's name can be taped to a board made for a specific need.
2. A drawer handle screwed to the board may be grasped by the user's free hand, to steady his position or prevent involuntary motion. Straps may also serve this purpose.
3. A narrow, long baking pan can be used for desserts, to make scooping up puddings easier.
4. Discarded plastic ice cream containers may be screwed to the board as a receptacle for any glass equipped with a straw.

For lunchroom purposes in a day-care center or other organization, a management chart, such as that used at the Day Care Center for CP Mentally Retarded, United Cerebral Palsy of Detroit, serves a valuable purpose in keeping track of each child's specific needs (Table 5-1).

## SELF-FEEDING AIDS FOR ADULTS

Aids to control motion when eating should be minimal and should only be used when the patient has been optimally seated for balance and position. A number of aids are available or can be devised to assist adults in self-feeding. Even a nonambulatory person with residual tonic neck reflex and very limited hand function can be positioned and supplied with eating aids that give some independence (Fig. 5-29).

1. A wheelchair insert will flex the trunk slightly forward to a normal position for eating. It also promotes good body alignment for sitting. Reclining or tilt-back positions for eating are contraindicated.
2. A seat belt over the lap and a cut-out tray at waist height avoid the need for bands around the chest. See Precautions for Seat Belts and Safety Supports in Chapter 1.
3. A flexion seat insert helps the patient to sit well back in the chair, to keep his weight on his buttocks and to reduce thrust.

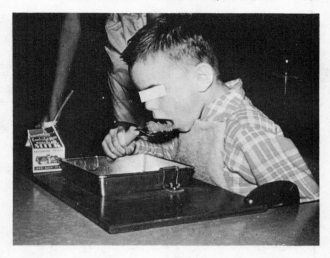

**FIG. 5-28.** Aluminum baking pan fastened to wood base to serve as dish. (Courtesy of A. Slominski, Cerebral Palsy Clinic, Indiana University Medical Center)

**FIG. 5-29.** Eating aids for severely disabled patient. Plate holder with well is tapered to facilitate sliding arm up board to reach the plate. Food guard holds food in place for easy lifting onto spoon. Patient is sipping from straw in container held in a wire beverage holder. (From Bensberg, G. J., ed. *Teaching the Mentally Retarded: A Handbook for Ward Personnel.* Atlanta, Southern Regional Education Board, 1966. Reproduced with permission)

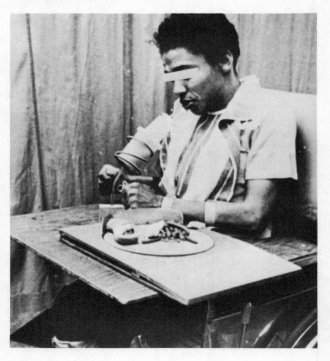

Table 5-1. Management Chart for Feeding Program in a Day Care Center

| Food portion | Feeding position | Method of eating | Hand preference | Chewing and swallowing | Sucking and drinking |
|---|---|---|---|---|---|
| Medium | Table-sitting, regular chair | Spoon with help | Right | No trouble | Glass with help |
| Small | Table sitting, arm chair | Spoon with help; finger feeds | Left | Eats bite-size or strained foods | Glass with help |
| Small | Relaxation chair | Dependent | Neither | Vernor's gingerale; fed mashed foods only | 2 bottles a day; cup or glass with help |
| Small | Table-sitting, regular chair | Independent, with spoon | Right | No trouble | Glass without help |
| Medium | Table-sitting, arm chair | Dependent | Neither | Some chewing difficulty; use strained, mashed, or soft foods | Training cup only |
| Small | High chair | Spoon with help; finger feeds | Left | No difficulty with mashed or strained foods | 2 bottles, A.M. and P.M.; cup with help |
| Small | Relaxation chair | Dependent | Neither | Eats strained or mashed foods | Does not drink juice; glass with straw |
| Medium | Table-sitting, regular chair | Dependent, with spoon | Right | No chewing difficulty | Straw, cup, glass, with help |
| Medium | Table-sitting, regular chair | Spoon with help | Right | Problem swallowing liquids; no chewing difficulty | Training cup |
| Small | Lying in Infa-Seat | Dependent | Neither | Eats strained or junior foods, fruits; problem swallowing | Bottle sometimes; sucking problem |
| Medium | Table-sitting, regular chair | Spoon with help | Right | Mashed or cut up, fine foods; problem with solids | Straw without help; cup or glass with help |
| Large | Table-sitting, regular chair | Independent with spoon | Right | No difficulty | Glass without help |
| Medium | Relaxation chair | Dependent | Left | Difficulty chewing and swallowing | Glass with straw; difficulty sucking; needs help |

Courtesy of the Day Care Center for CP Mentally Retarded, United Cerebral Palsy of Detroit.

4. A firm footrest will assure stabilization which frees residual arm function.
5. Use of a straw for drinking helps to promote lip control and fosters swallowing with the head upright.
6. A wire, patio-type beverage holder can be cut to a height that enables the patient to reach the glass or cup and can be inserted into a wood block to hold it in position.
7. A cockup splint on the patient's arm can facilitate holding a spoon or fork.
8. A plate guard helps the patient to get food onto a spoon or fork.
9. A plate holder of wood, with a cut-out "well" stabilizes the plate, and it can be made with a tapered edge to help the patient slide his arm up to the plate.

## WRIST AND ANKLE WEIGHTS TO CONTROL MOTION

Wrist and ankle weights of soft black leatherette filled with tiny lead pellets are available (Fig. 5-30). The weights can be easily molded to body contours and quickly attached by means of a Velcro fastener. Accessory extension pieces are also available to allow multiple use. Specify whether they are to be for adult or child use. Special sizes and shapes can be supplied on request.

### Source

Cleo Living Aids

## ARM CONTROL STRAP

An arm control strap helps a patient with flailing motion to bring his arm to midline (Fig. 5-31). Such straps are useful on a child with involuntary motion at the shoulders or one who holds one or both arms abducted, as in asymmetrical tonic neck reflex. The straps can be used instead of wrist weights and sometimes work better. They are also helpful for the child who hits himself or others involuntarily or for one who catches his arms in doors. Straps can be worn at the wrist, or on one wrist and one upper arm; usually, however, they are worn on both upper arms.

### Construction

An arm-control strap consists of 3 parts: the first part goes around arm or wrist of the wearer; the sec-

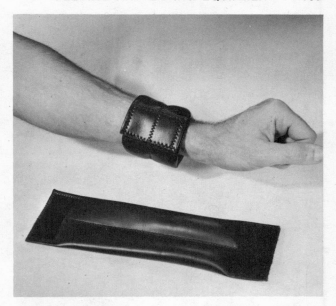

**FIG. 5-30.** Weighted wrist cuff to control motion. (Courtesy of Cleo Living Aids, Cleveland, Ohio)

**FIG. 5-31.** Arm straps to help control involuntary shoulder motion or arm abduction. (Courtesy of P. Holser-Buehler, United Cerebral Palsy Association of Los Angeles County)

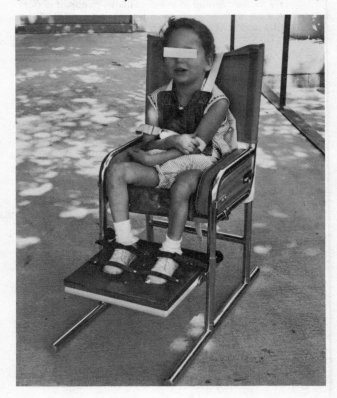

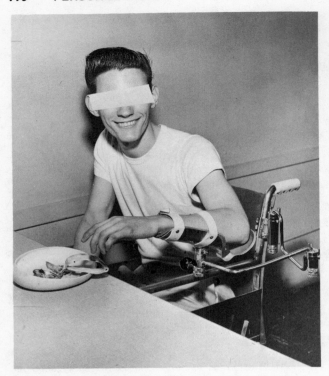

**FIG. 5-32.** Upper extremity control brace, to help control involuntary motion. Suited to many patient's needs, it is often useful as a therapeutic training aid, enabling patient to discontinue its use, once an activity is learned. (Courtesy of P. Holser Buehler, United Cerebral Palsy Association of Los Angeles County) AJOT 16:170–175, July–Aug., 1962

ond part is elastic and is held by D rings to the first and the third part; and the third part is like the first and can be buckled onto the wearer's other arm or wrist.

1. Use 1-inch webbing long enough to span each upper arm, with allowance for a 1-inch foldover for a buckle and a ½-inch foldover for a D ring. (This ranges between 8 and 12 inches.) Use 1-inch elastic webbing about 5–7 inches long, including fold over, for middle section, D rings may be 1-inch or ½-inch size.
2. Sew a two-prong buckle to one end of webbing.
3. Sew a D ring or metal curtain ring directly below the buckle.
4. Repeat procedure on second piece of webbing.
5. Elastic webbing is doubled between the two D rings. Adjust the elastic to hold the arms in the midline but still permit the child some range of motion. Sew in place.

## ARM CONTROL BRACE

This brace (Fig. 5-32) aids in the control of involuntary motion of the arm. It may be used with the severely involved patient to teach the use of the spelling board, a step toward typing and other arm activities. It has proved valuable with the moderately involved athetoid for learning self-feeding, typing, drawing, painting, and writing. It serves as a therapeutic training aid since the use of the control brace may be discontinued once the activity is learned.

### Source

Orthopedic Supplies Co.

### Mechanics of Construction

The mechanism of the control brace is illustrated in Figures 5-33, 5-34, and 5-35.

1. Two $\frac{7}{16}$-inch stainless steel rods are welded to three movable friction joints (A, B, and C, Fig. 5-34), which permit the arm to move in a horizontal plane.
2. An arm trough with an elbow support, into which the patient's arm is strapped, is attached by a fourth friction joint (D) to the terminal friction joint (C). Joint D permits the patient to move his arm in the vertical plane. All four friction joints can be tightened in any degree to give resistance to motion.
3. Stops located on the two proximal joints, A and B, are adjustable with an Allen wrench to restrict range of motion when desired.
4. The distal rod (B to C) is bent 60 degrees toward the midline to permit free excursion of the arm trough and brings it closer to the body. The bent rod creates a control brace for right- or left-handed use which cannot be interchanged.
5. A brace fits into a bracket (X, Fig. 5-35), which can be mounted to the upright on the back of the wheelchair or, with modifications, to a straight-backed chair. The bracket, into which the brace slips, is angled about 10 degrees forward into the vertical plane. When it is rotated parallel to the upright of the wheelchair, it lowers the height of the brace at its most terminal part and corrects the back angle of the wheelchair upright.

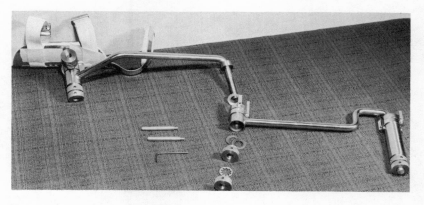

**FIG. 5-33.** Components of upper extremity control brace. (Courtesy of P. Holser-Buehler, United Cerebral Palsy Association of Los Angeles County)

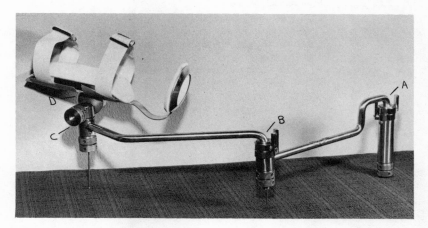

**FIG. 5-34.** Structure of upper extremity control brace. Three movable friction joints, *A, B,* and *C.* Arm trough is attached with fourth friction joint, *D.* (Courtesy of P. Holser-Buehler, United Cerebral Palsy Association of Los Angeles County)

**FIG. 5-35.** Upper extremity control brace fastened to chair back with angled bracket, *X.* (Courtesy of P. Holser-Buehler, United Cerebral Palsy Association of Los Angeles County)

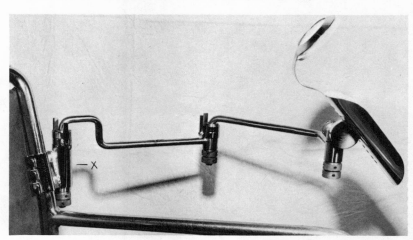

# REFERENCES

### Sucking Aids

Haynes, U. H. "Nursing approaches in cerebral dysfunction," Am J Nurs, Vol 68:10, 2170–2176, Oct. 1968.

### Positioning for Feeding

Bensberg, G. J., ed. *Teaching the Mentally Retarded: A Handbook for Ward Personnel.* Atlanta, Southern Regional Educational Board, 1966.

Denhoff, E., Langdon, M., eds. "Cerebral dysfunction: a treatment program for young children." Clin Pediat 5:332, 1966. (See particularly the speech section.)

Finnie, N. R., *Handling The Young Cerebral Palsied at Home.* New York, Dutton and Company, Inc., 1970.

### Self-Feeding Aids

"Before and After of Two Athetoids Using the Upper Extremity Control Brace." United Cerebral Palsy Association of Los Angeles County, Van Nuys, Calif. (16 mm. movie)

Danzig, A. L. *A Handbook for One-Handers,* New York, Federation of the Handicapped, 1957.

American Occupational Therapy Association, Ed. "Feeding suggestions for the training of the cerebral palsied." Am J Occup Ther 7:19, 1953. (Reprint available from the United Cerebral Palsy Associations, Inc., New York.)

New York Univ. Medical Center, Ed. *Self-Help Devices for Rehabilitation,* Dubuque, Iowa, Vol. I, 1958, Vol. II, 1965.

Holser, P. *Upper Extremity Control Brace—Instruction Manual.* New York, American Occupational Therapy Association.

Holser, P., Jones, M., Ilanit, T. "A study of the upper extremity control brace," Am J Occup Ther 16:170–175, 1962.

Klinger, J., Frieden, F., Sullivan, R., *Mealtime Manual for the Aged and Handicapped.* New York, Simon & Schuster, 1970.

Leon, H. E., Cohen, P. "An arm restrainer for the athetoid," Am J Occup Ther 8:204, 1950.

Nathen, C., Slominski, A., Griswold, P. *Please Help Us Help Ourselves—Inexpensive Adapted Equipment for the Handicapped,* Indianapolis, Manual, Occupational Therapy Dept. at Indiana University Medical Center, 1970.

### Professional Guides

ICTA Information Centre, Bromma, Sweden.

"Self-Help Devices for Handicapped: Bibliography." National Easter Seal Society for Crippled Children and Adults.

Lowman, E., Klinger, J. *Aids to Independent Living—Self Help for the Handicapped.* New York, McGraw-Hill, 1967.

# 6
# Special Clothing and Dressing Aids

Clothing and dressing aids are presented from two aspects: What will be useful for the person who is caring for the disabled person to know, and what will help the disabled individual to care for himself as independently as possible.

## MEASURING TO ASSURE CORRECT SIZE

As with equipment, measurement is the first step in obtaining suitable clothing fit. Proper fit is necessary for comfort, as well as for appearance, which can be a help to morale. Since individual needs of disabled persons are likely to vary widely, it is advisable to consult special sources of information on clothing adaptations so that deformities such as marked scoliosis can be taken into account. A shoulder that is much higher than the other or a hip that is higher and/or wider will greatly affect fit. A number of information sources are given in the References section of this chapter. The measuring instructions given below are standard techniques. In all instances, for outer garments, measurements should be made over the clothing which will be worn beneath.

**FIG. 6-1.** Measuring child's height, chest, waist, and hips. (After photos of measurement, Sears Roebuck and Company, Chicago, Ill.)

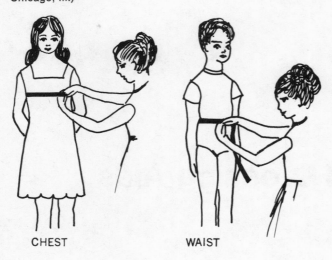

CHEST          WAIST

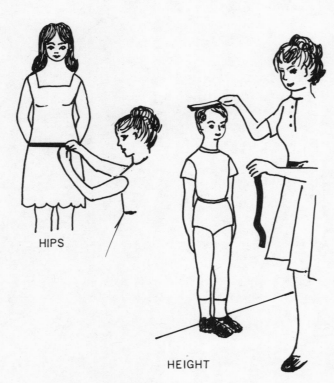

HIPS          HEIGHT

## CHILDREN'S MEASURING INSTRUCTIONS

1. Height. This is the most important measurement for determining size (Fig. 6-1). Be sure to measure without shoes. Have child stand against the wall, if he is able, and make a mark level with the top of the head. Measure from this point down to the floor.
2. Chest. Use a tape measure around the body at the fullest part of the chest. Hold the tape firm but not tight. Be sure the tape is straight across the back, and that the child is standing naturally.
3. Waist. Measure around the smallest part of the natural waistline. Hold the tape firm but not tight. When measuring for slacks, pants, or shorts, measure over shirt with the tape at the height at which the garment will be worn.
4. Hips. Child should be standing naturally and his feet should be together in a natural position. Measure in a straight line around the body at the fullest part of the hips.
5. Inseam. See Men's Measuring Instructions below.
6. Length. For full-length garments, measure from collar line at the back of the neck to bottom edge that garment is to reach. Length to waistline is a useful measure to have. For skirt, measure side back from waistline to hemline.
7. Headwear. Measure around the head above the ears. If the measurement is between sizes, you should order the next size larger.
8. Variations to note. General build should be considered. Height is the deciding factor when a child's height and weight fall into different sizes. To determine whether his size is Slim, Regular, or Husky, check his weight (in his underwear) in that size. For example, a size 11 child, 56 inches tall, would be considered Slim if his weight were 72 pounds, Regular if his weight were 80 pounds, or Husky if his weight were 88 pounds.

## MEN'S MEASURING INSTRUCTIONS

1. Chest. Measure around the chest, well up under the arms and across the shoulder blades (Fig. 6-2, *A*). Hold the tape firm and level; be sure it does not slip down in back.
2. Height. Measurement should be taken from the top of the head to the floor while individual is standing in stocking feet with heels against the wall. Sizes are designated by letters: *S* (short), 5 feet 3 inches to 5 feet 7 inches; *R* (regular), over 5 feet 7 inches to 5 feet 11 inches; *T* (tall), over 5 feet 11 inches to 6 feet 3 inches; *XT* (extra tall), over 6 feet 3

inches to 6 feet 7 inches. On garments, these sizes are usually indicated by letters after the chest or inseam measurement.

3. Waist. Measure over shirt, not over trousers (Fig. 6-2, *B*) at position where trousers or slacks are normally worn. Hold the tape firm but not tight.

4. Inseam. If a pair of well-fitting slacks of the style you wish to purchase is available, lay them flat on a table. Fold back one leg (Fig. 6-2, *C*) and measure along the inseam from the crotch seam to the bottom of the cuff.

5. Outseam. Measure from waist to ankle (or bottom of trouser cuff along side seam).

6. Sleeve. If a specific length is required, bend the elbow and measure from the middle of the back of the neck, across the shoulder and around the point of the elbow to the wrist (Fig. 6-2, *D*).

7. Neck. Measure around the middle of the neck, or lay the collar of a well-fitting shirt flat and measure from the center of the collar button to the far end of the buttonhole (Fig. 6-2, *E*).

8. Headwear. Measured in the same way as for children.

9. Gloves. Place tape measure around the fullest part of the hand over the knuckles, with the hand flat, not including the thumb. Fingers should be together. Measure the hand usually used—right for the right-handed person, left for the left-handed. The number of inches will determine the size.

## WOMEN'S MEASURING INSTRUCTIONS

Measurements should be taken carefully over whatever type of foundation garments the individual will wear (Figs. 6-3 and 6-4).

1. Bust. Measure around the fullest part (Fig. 6-3, 1), keeping the tape straight in back.

2. Chest. Place tape well up under the arms, above the bust.

3. Waist. Measure at the smallest part (Fig. 6-3, 2), holding tape firm but not tight.

4. Hips. Measure around the fullest part (Fig. 6-3, 3), keeping feet together and holding the tape firm and being sure it is level around the hips.

5. Length. For dresses and other full-length garments, measure from point of prominent neck bone at the back of the neck to bottom edge of hemline desired. For skirts, girdles, etc., measure from waist down side back to hemline desired.

6. Rise. Measure from waist at center front, down through the crotch and up to the waist at center back (Fig. 6-4).

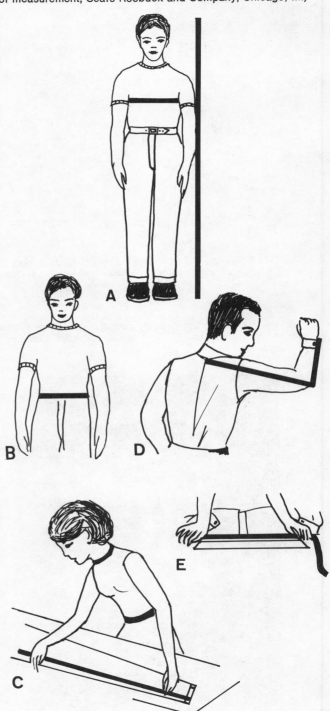

**FIG. 6-2.** Measuring man's chest and height, *A;* waist, *B;* inseam of slacks, *C;* sleeve, *D;* and collar, *E.* (After photos of measurement, Sears Roebuck and Company, Chicago, Ill.)

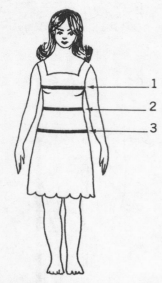

**FIG. 6-3.** Measuring woman's bust, 1; waist, 2; and hips, 3. (After photos of measurement, Sears Roebuck and Company, Chicago)

**FIG. 6-4.** Measuring chest, bust, waist, hips, and rise. (After photos of measurement, Sears Roebuck and Company, Chicago).

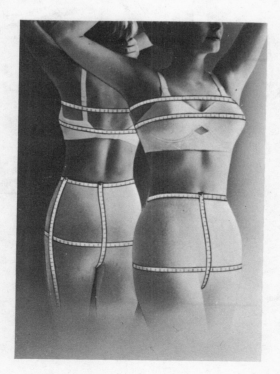

## SELECTING SIZES

Pattern manufacturers have adopted standard sizing, and key measurements appear on all patterns. If garments are going to be made for the physically disabled, a basic pattern would be of great value. All necessary alterations and adjustments can be made on the muslin basic pattern so that all future garment patterns can be altered in the initial stages of laying out the pattern and cutting. New adjustments would have to be made periodically, however, for major weight changes or for the rapidly growing child.

In ready-made garments, the size markings on store racks are not dependable, varying widely among the manufacturers, and measurements should be verified before purchasing such clothing. In selecting clothes for purchase in the store or by mail order, observe the following guidelines that are based on the proper measurements taken according to the instructions given above.

### HATS

The size is the number of inches determined in the measurement.

### GLOVES

The size is the number of inches measured around the hand.

### SHORTS, SLACKS, AND SKIRTS

Choose the size closest to the hip measurement.

### TROUSERS AND SLACKS

For men and boys choose the size closest to the waist measurement and length.

### SHIRTS

For men and boys, choose according to collar size and sleeve length.

For women and girls, select the size closest to the bust measurement.

### JACKETS AND COATS

For men and boys, select the size closest to the chest measurement.

For women and girls, select the size closest to the bust measurement.

## ROBES AND LOUNGEWEAR

Choose size closest to chest measurement for men and boys, and bust measurement for women and girls.

## SWEATERS

For men and boys, choose the size closest to chest measurement, plus 3 to 4 inches.

For women and girls, choose the size by bust measurement, in accordance with the following chart:

| Bust (inches) | Sweater size |
|---|---|
| 30½–32 | 34 |
| 32½–34 | 36 |
| 34½–36 | 38 |
| 36½–38 | 40 |
| 38½–40 | 42 |
| 40½–42 | 44 |
| 42½–44 | 46 |

## BLOUSES

For junior sizes, select the size closest to the bust measurement. For misses' and women's sizes, choose the size according to the following chart:

| Bust (inches) | Sweater size |
|---|---|
| 28½–30 | 30 |
| 30½–32 | 32 |
| 32½–34 | 34 |
| 34½–36 | 36 |
| 36½–38 | 38 |
| 38½–40 | 40 |
| 40½–42 | 42 |
| 42½–44 | 44 |

## SHEATH DRESSES AND SUITS

Choose the size closest to the hip measurement.

## MATERNITY FASHIONS

Choose according to prematernity size. Expansion is allowed by adjustable waists or stretch fronts.

## BRASSIERES

Select by chest measurement. To determine cup size, subtract chest measurement from bust measurement. The difference, in inches, will indicate the proper cup size: *AAA*, bust the same as or less than chest; *AA*, bust up to ½ inch larger than chest; *A*, bust ½ inch up to 1½ inches larger; *B*, bust over 1½ inches up to 2½ inches larger; *C*, bust over 2½ inches up to 3½ inches larger; *D*, bust over 3½ inches up to 4½ inches larger; *DD*, bust over 4½ up to 5½ inches larger; *F*, bust slightly fuller than a *DD* cup.

Some women find brassieres with self-straps more comfortable to wear (Fig. 6-5) and those with front openings easier to put on.

## GIRDLES, PANTY GIRDLES, AND BRIEFS

Select according to waist measurement, but be sure that hip, length, and rise will also be correct. For all-in-one foundations, select by bra size and then make sure that other measurements will be correct.

**FIG. 6-5.** Brassieres with self straps (*A*) and front closure (*B*). (Courtesy of Sears Roebuck and Company, Chicago)

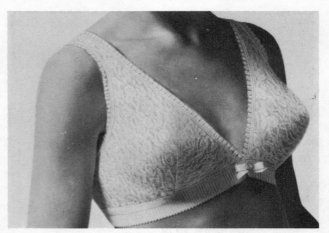

A

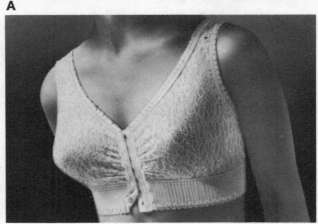

B

# SPECIALLY DESIGNED CLOTHES FOR ADULTS

### VGRS DESIGNS FOR WOMEN

Within its own caseload the Rehabilitation Center of Vocational Guidance and Rehabilitation Services (VGRS) sees a daily need for clothing that is easy to put on, affords comfort, meets various physical needs and is attractive. They are frequently asked to assist in meeting special clothing needs in addition to their other rehabilitation services.

Since they have a sewing workroom in which they employ some of their clients who have been skillfully trained in sewing, they began to produce useful and helpful clothing ideas. As a result, they were asked to expand and offer these designs nationally. After consulting with manufacturers and stores, they decided that the services could be offered most practically by mail order. New items are added continuously.

Attractive, smooth-fitting Bermuda shorts (Fig. 6-6), styled for action, are one example of their offerings. Velcro tape on both side seams makes the shorts easy to put on. An adjustable back waistband and an inner belt keep the shorts in position and easy to fasten. Made of minimum-care sturdy cotton blends, the shorts come in beige, chocolate, gray, light and dark blue, gold, pastel pink, and yellow.

Another item is the quality tailored slip (Fig. 6-7), full-length, with front opening—which means no more over-the-head donning! The slip is made of fine dacron and cotton broadcloth, and has built-up shoulders and gentle bust-line darts. It comes in white, light blue, and pink. It is also available with a terry back panel, or with embroidery trimming.

Among other VGRS designs available are: all-occasion ensemble, all-occasion dress, all-weather coat, wrapper back dress, shoulder shrug, easy-on robe, half slip, adjustable flared skirt, tailored blouse, women's slacks, exercise skirt, and therapy shorts.

### Source for VGRS Designs

Vocational Guidance and Rehabilitation Services

### Another Source for Women's Clothing

Clothing Research and Development Foundation (functional fashions)

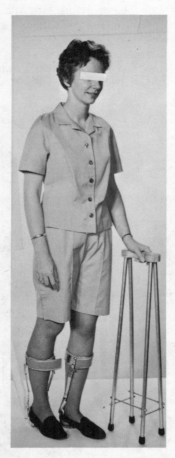

**FIG. 6-6.** Bermuda shorts, specially designed to put on with ease. (Courtesy of Vocational Guidance and Rehabilitation Services, Cleveland, Ohio)

## WHEELCHAIR CAPE

A cape suitable for wheelchair users was designed at the New York University Medical Center, Institute of Rehabilitation Medicine, as part of a clothing research project. It is not available commercially.

Made of warm wool zibeline, the cape can be worn over anything, as it closes all the way up the front with Velcro and keeps everything underneath hidden from view. The collar turns well up to keep the neck warm. It may be styled for women (Fig. 6-8) or men (Fig. 6-9).

This cape was found particularly useful by therapists at the Spastic Aid of Alabama for uncontrolled young adult athetoids for whom an inexpensive variation was made by using government surplus alpaca cloth.

### Instructions

The idea of using a cape, a velcro closure, and a high neck can be applied to any cape pattern.

### SPECIAL SLACKS FOR MEN

Full-length side-seam zipper on both legs of these slacks open all the way from bottom up, or all the way from top down, or half way. The slacks have concealed zippers, a roomy seat for wheelchair ease, and full front lining to resist wear by braces. A half-belt of trouser material buttons inside to hold the front and the back of the trousers so that they will not drop to the floor while being zipped.

### Source of Information for Men's Clothing

Clothing Research and Development Foundation

## SPECIAL SELF-HELP CLOTHES FOR CHILDREN

The selection of comfortable, attractive clothing that a child can manage is an important part of his development and rehabilitation. His clothing should be functional to encourage independence in dressing and to give him confidence in doing for himself (Fig. 6-10). What do you buy to meet his need? There is no simple answer, but it may help to keep the following ideas in mind while shopping.

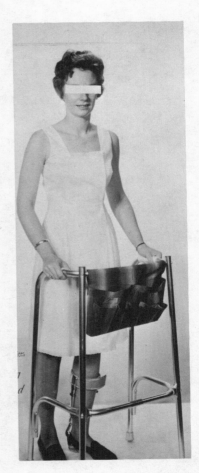

**FIG. 6-7.** Slip with front opening, easy to get into. (Courtesy of Vocational Guidance and Rehabilitation Services, Cleveland, Ohio)

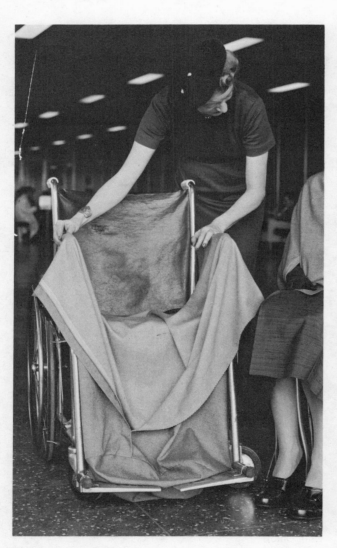

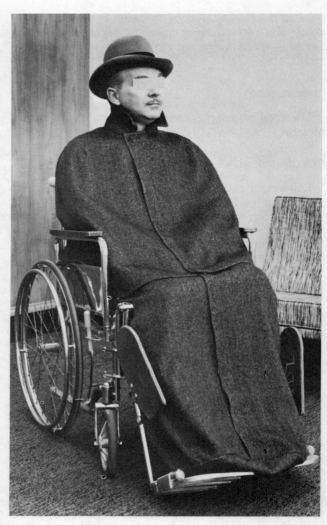

**FIG. 6-8.** Wheelchair cape. (Courtesy of the Institute of Rehabilitation Medicine, New York University Medical Center)

**FIG. 6-9.** Wheelchair cape for man. (Courtesy of the Institute of Rehabilitation Medicine, New York University Medical Center)

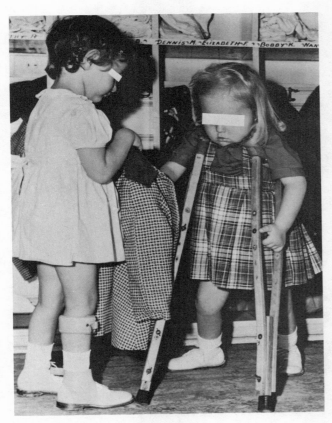

**FIG. 6-10.** Wide raglan sleeve of coat, making it easy for child to slip on. (Courtesy of the National Society of Crippled Children and Adults, Chicago, Ill.)

1. Select simple lines and cuts that are attractive and allow extra room for body movement.
2. Select clothes that are easy to take off and put on.
3. Select openings and fasteners that are within easy reach and grasp of the child.
4. Select fabrics that do not wrinkle or show spots or stains readily.
5. Select clothes with fabric interest—color combinations, prints, or checks—rather than fussy details.
6. Know your child's measurements and buy clothes that are sized for his needs.

## SELF-HELP FEATURES

In selecting children's clothes so that they may help themselves, there are several features to be checked.
1. Easy openings for garments, such as full-length center front opening; large or expandable neck openings for over-the-head donning; easy-to-grasp and easy-to-reach openings
2. Raglan or kimono sleeves, which allow freedom of movement
3. Easily identified front and back
4. Long thread shanks on buttons (Fig. 6-11)
5. Gripper fasteners (Fig. 6-11) that are at least standard size (about the size of a dime), if they do not fit too tightly together.
6. Large metal hooks (Fig. 6-11), such as those used on the waistbands of trousers, that are easy for a child to manipulate.
7. Velcro fasteners

### Sources

Vocational Guidance and Rehabilitation Services
Clothing Research and Development Foundation

**FIG. 6-11.** *Left,* long thread shank on buttons for easy closure. *Right, top,* grippers; *bottom,* large hook easy for child to manipulate. (From Boettke, E. *Suggestions for Physically Handicapped Mothers on Clothing for Preschool Children.* Storrs, Conn., Research Center, School of Home Economics, University of Connecticut, 1958. Reproduced with permission)

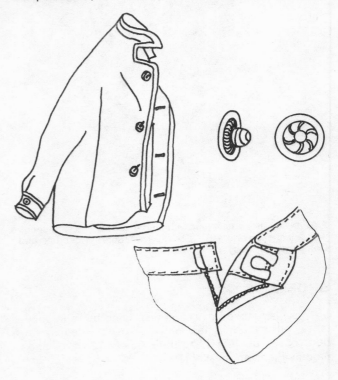

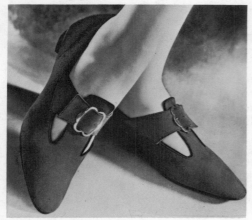

**A**

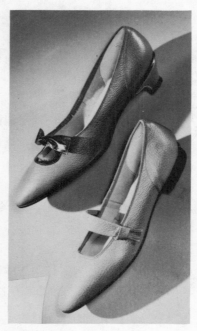

**B**

**FIG. 6-12.** Shoes fastened with single buckle (*A*), and shoes with elastic inserts (*B*). (Courtesy of Sears Roebuck and Company, Chicago)

## SHOE AIDS

There is no need to spend time tying bows in shoelaces, particularly when they can become easily untied, constituting a hazard to safety. Several shoe modifications are available

### TALON SHUN-LOKS

This zipper shoe fastener can be adapted to any size laced shoe. It comes with full instructions for installation by a local shoemaker.

**Source**

Fred Sammons, Inc.

### ELASTIC SHOE LACES

Elastic shoe laces eliminate lacing by allowing the shoes to be slipped on or off without tying or untying.

**Sources**

J. A. Preston Corp. (Flex-O-Lace)
Rehab Aids (Elastie)

### OTHER SHOE AIDS

Shoes with a single simple buckle or elastic inserts (Fig. 6-12) are easy to put on and take off, provide good support, and can be good-looking shoes.

**Source**

Sears Roebuck and Co.

### SHOE AND GLOVE SIZE INFORMATION EXCHANGE

For help in contacting persons with odd shoes or gloves available, write to Amputee Shoe and Glove Exchange, c/o Dr. and Mrs. Richard E. Wainerdi.

## GARTERLESS HOSE

To eliminate the need for garters, which may impede circulation, or of supporters, which may be uncomfortable, knee-length stretch-top socks are available for men, women, and children. Some types of over-the-knee stockings also have elastic stretch tops (Fig. 6-13). Mesh hose have more stretch. Pantyhose or tights also eliminate garters. For comfort and protection against irritation, it is advisable to use some form of panty, however, small, beneath pantyhose. And here is a good tip: It is easier to get into nylon hose and pantyhose if the wearer first puts on a pair of nylon Peds.

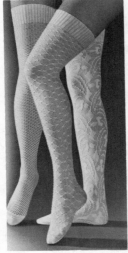

**A**

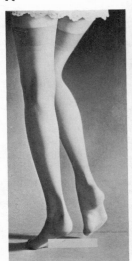

**B**

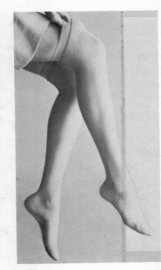

**C**

**FIG. 6-13.** Hose with elastic tops (*A, B,* and *C*). (Courtesy of Sears Roebuck and Company, Chicago)

### Source

Sears Roebuck and Co. (Local Stores)

## VELCRO TAPE

The Velcro Tape (Fig. 6-14) used for the closure on the wheelchair cape and on other garments described in this chapter can be used for many types of clothing, and has a great many other uses as well (several examples appear throughout this manual). There are no moving parts to the closure, the tape cannot snag, and it opens at a touch. It grips with two surfaces of nylon tape that adhere to each other securely, yet open quickly and easily from either end. Velcro can be dry-cleaned or washed but should never be ironed with a hot iron.

### Pointer

To form a joint between hook and loop Velcro without sewing, the following procedure is suggested. Flood a ½-inch area of hook with cement (Velcro, Duco, Barge, etc.). Engage the loop portion firmly into the cement and the hooks and allow to dry overnight. The resultant joint will be neat and strong.

### Source

Smalley & Bates, Inc.

## USEFUL GADGETS

### APRON CLIP

An apron clip makes an apron easy to get into and out of in seconds without having to reach around the back. The clip is made of plastic, is unbreakable, and clips around the waist to hold the apron in place. With

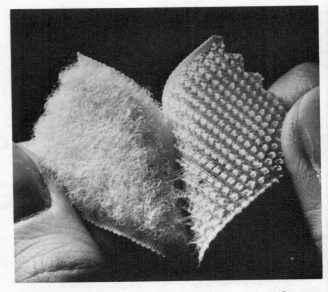

**FIG. 6-14.** Velcro tape, showing gripping surfaces. (Courtesy of Smalley & Bates, Inc., New York)

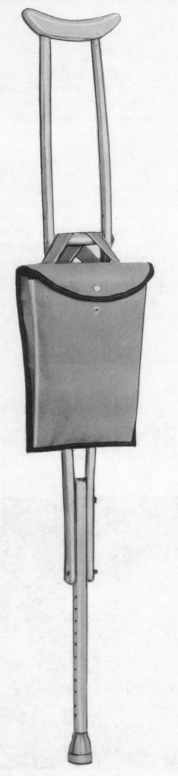

an apron clip, any woman can make an apron in minutes. The clip is easily slipped into or out of the apron, allowing the apron to be ironed flat. The clip comes on a card with complete easy-to-follow instructions for making an apron.

**Sources**

Cleo Living Aids
Vocational Guidance and Rehabilitation Services

## UTILITY CRUTCH BAG

A useful crutch bag (Fig. 6-15) has been designed for the crutch user, whose hands are not free to manage a purse or briefcase.

**Sources**

J. A. Preston Corp.
Cleo Living Aids
Vocational Guidance and Rehabilitation Services

## BUTTON AIDS

For a person with limited dexterity, a button aid facilitates fastening buttons (Fig. 6-16). The three most useful models are one with a regular handle, one with a knob handle, and one with a rubber handle. The aid comes with instructions for use.

**Source**

Fred Sammons, Inc.

## MAGNETS

Magnetic bars or strips fastened to walls, work tables, or the inside of closets hold in place an array of items from steel wool to sewing equipment. Magnetized tools can be fastened to metal cabinets or other equipment.

Magnetic shields, bars, disks, and stripping can be fastened to wheelchairs, beds, or stand-in tables, tractions, crutches, casts, or even to the patient himself (e.g., magnetic wrist or finger band) and thereby facilitate availability and manipulation of tools or materials. Just to mention one potential: A patient with loss of finger sensation would be able to sew without exaggerated pinching force to hold the needle if flexible magnetic tape (available in 1-inch width) were placed, thimble fashion, around the thumb and forefinger. The attraction of magnetic tape is not strong enough to pull the needle back out of the material.

Under specific circumstances a magnetic device could aid a patient with poor hand grasp. The visually handicapped and the aged could also profit from "magnetic assistance." In homemaking and household tasks, magnetized devices could be assistive in many situations, since it is easier to put an object against a surface than on a hook.

Alnico and ceramic magnets in any shape or form are readily available for reasonable prices in hardware shops, dime stores, discount houses, magazine shopping guides, or through catalogs intended for school sciences, industry, and hobbyists.

The Edmund Scientific Co. offers lode stones and gap-magnets to do your own magnetizing and reloading, but any high school science department would surely be glad to make this its project.

## LEFT-HANDED SCISSORS

There are three kinds of left-handed scissors:

1. In the conventional type, the blades are fastened so that the blade with the top handle is toward the right, or inside, for the left-handed person. He can force the blades together by pushing the handles out as he cuts. These are available either in children's scissors, with both handles of equal size, or in shears, with one handle larger for the fingers.
2. In this type, the blades are in the same relationship as those in right-handed scissors (i.e., the top handle is to the left), but the handle for the thumb is shaped differently so that it conforms comfortably when the thumb is inserted from the left or outside. Some left-handed people find this type of scissors easier to use than the conventional left-handed scissors.
3. This type, usually scissors and not shears, is exactly like right-handed scissors, except that the word "lefty" or "left-handed" is printed on one blade. Since bona fide left-handed scissors may also have these words impressed on the blade, purchasers should be wary and examine the scissors before deciding to buy.

**FIG. 6-16.** Seven button aids with easy hand grips. (Courtesy of Fred Sammons, Inc., Brookfield, Ill.)

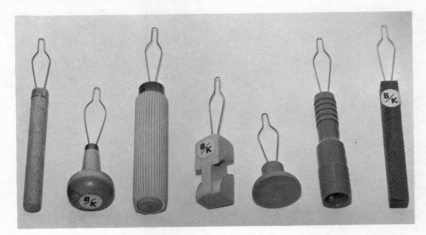

# REFERENCES

### Special Clothing

Bare, C., Boettke, E., Waggoner, N. *Self-Help Clothing for Handicapped Children*. Chicago, National Easter Seal Society for Crippled Children and Adults. (Guide for parents and professional personnel in selecting children's clothes and in adapting them to make use of as much independence as the child can manage.)

Boettke, E. "Suggestions for Physically Handicapped Mothers on Clothing for Preschool Children," Research Center, School of Home Economics, University of Connecticut." (Features self-help, growth, wear, easy care of clothing.)

Danzig, A. L. *Handbook for One-Handers*. New York, Federation of the Handicapped, 1957.

"Dressing Techniques for the Cerebral Palsied Child," United Cerebral Palsy Associations, Inc., (Suggestions from a group of occupational therapists for clothing adaptations, fasteners, and self-help aids.)

"Flexible Fashions," Superintendent of Documents, U.S. Government Printing Office, Washington, D.C. (Clothing adaptations for the woman with arthritis: outer and under garments and fastenings. Included are purchasing suggestions and sources of functional clothing.)

"Functionally Designed Clothing Aids for Chronically Ill and Disabled," Rehabilitation Services Administration, U.S. Department of Health, Education, and Welfare, Washington, D.C.

Hall, D. S., Vignos, P. J. "Clothing Adaptations," Am J Occup Ther 18:108, 1964.

Hallenbeck, P. "Special Clothing for the Handicapped; Review of Research & Resources," Rehab Lit; 27:2:34–40, Feb. 1966.

May, E., Waggoner, N., and Boettke, E. "Selection and Adaptation of Clothing to Suit Particular Needs for Men, Women and Children," From *Homemaking for the Handicapped*. New York, Dodd Mead, 1966. (See also chapters on "Self-Help Clothing for Adults" and "Self-Help Clothing for Children.")

Scott, C. "Clothes for the Physically Handicapped Homemaker," Clothing and Housing Research Report No. 12, 1962.

### Magnets

Hardy, L. "Magnets," AOTA Bulletin on Practice 2:4, Dec. 1967.

### Left-Handed Scissors

Mullin, E., and Price, A. "AOTA Bulletin on Practice," 2:4, Sept. 1967.

### Professional Guides

ICTA Information Centre, Bromma, Sweden.

"Self-Help Devices for the Handicapped: Bibliography," Library, National Easter Seal Society for Crippled Children and Adults.

"Self-Help Devices for Rehabilitation: Arthritis Self-Help Devices," New York University Medical Center, Institute of Rehabilitation Medicine.

Cookman, H. and Zimmerman, M. "Functional Fashions for the Physically Handicapped," New York University Medical Center, Institute of Rehabilitation Medicine, Patient Publication III, 1971.

# 7
# Personal Hygiene Aids

Personal hygiene goes further than mere cleanliness. It involves the type of fastidious care that is required of adults in a highly competitive society. Some people need special aids to help with the simplest tasks. Others need to recognize that outsiders, who may be willing to look upon their abilities rather than their disabilities, are often not willing to be subjected to lacks of personal hygiene.

The disabled individual should ask the following questions of himself. If he cannot do so, perhaps his parent, teacher, or counselor may take the initiative.

Does a daily bath satisfy your needs? Or does the amount of exertion that you must expend make it also useful for you to use deodorants, lightly perfumed powders, and/or faintly scented toilet water?

When you smile, do clean teeth greet your listener? Or should you see a dentist and ask how to maintain your teeth in good order after he has fixed them for you?

When you whisper or talk directly at someone who is near, is your breath pleasant, or does it smell of neglected and unbrushed teeth?

Do you wear clean underclothing daily?

How often do you have to shave in order to look neat in the afternoon, when you are on an all-day job?

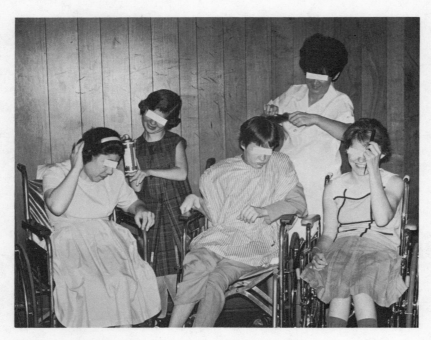

**FIG. 7-1.** Hair care for members of a UCP charm class. A hair stylist has helped each girl achieve a becoming style. Angelina, at left, has naturally curly hair. Keeping it cut short and using a hair band and spray means combing only once a day. Lorie has an "uncurly" permanent, which falls easily into soft waves. Priscilla's attractive short bob can be smoothed into place with one hand and needs little combing. Mary's bob is not so short, but she can comb the swirl into place using only her left hand. (Courtesy of United Cerebral Palsy of Philadelphia and Vicinity)

**FIG. 7-2.** Standard electric razors with hand-holds attached. (Courtesy of Fred Sammons, Inc., Brookfield, Ill.)

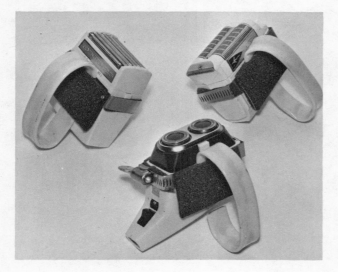

If hairs grow on your neck or face, have you checked with your doctor about the possibility of their removal?

Is your hair cut and shaped in a way that takes minimal care during the day? Is it easily washed often enough to have a clean shine?

Are your nails clean and neatly trimmed?

Are you the fellow who needs a T-shirt type of undershirt of cotton to keep perspiration off your shirt?

Are you the girl who needs shields to protect your dress from perspiration?

## GOOD GROOMING AIDS FOR YOUNG ADULTS

Careful attention to the details pointed out by the above list of questions will not only make the young adult more acceptable to others, but will help to increase poise and self-respect. A few helpful hints are given here.

### HAIR CARE FOR WOMEN

1. A young woman will often find that a good hair stylist can assist her in achieving an attractive style, requiring little attention during the day. If the style is simple, she may then be able to take care of it herself, with only an occasional visit to the stylist for a haircut or, perhaps, a permanent wave (Fig. 7-1).

2. An inexpensive washable wig might help to solve some emergency dilemmas in hair care.

3. Instead of bobby pins or barrettes to hold unruly hair in place, small combs often are easier to handle. Some come with gripper teeth to keep them in place.

## DRESS SHIELDS

Some women cannot obtain adequate protection from underarm moisture with antiperspirants. Dress shields will meet this need and protect the clothing from undue wear. The shields that come attached to a brassiere-like unit are most useful for this purpose because they can rinsed out after each wearing. They are available at drugstores, notion counters of department stores, or from catalog companies.

## ELECTRIC SHAVERS

Regular razors may prove to be a hazard for the handicapped person. Standard electric shavers can be used if adapted for easy handling. A hand strap is available that can be attached to a shaver, facilitating its use (Fig. 7-2).

### Source

Fred Sammons, Inc.

## SHOE SHINING EQUIPMENT

It need not take a great deal of "elbow grease" to have clean and shining shoes. Some types of electric shoe shiners can be easily used by the disabled individual. One has a hand strap to hold the unit while applying polish and giving a shine (Fig. 7-3). (This unit is also adaptable for other polishing jobs that might be undertaken.) The other unit requires only a tap of the toe to start and stop (Fig. 7-4).

### Source

Sears Roebuck and Co.

## BATHING EQUIPMENT

It is well known that the greatest number of home accidents occur in the bathroom. This being the case, more than usual care must be exerted to assure the safety of the handicapped person during bathing. There are a number of ingenious safeguards for the bather and some useful items for comfort and con-

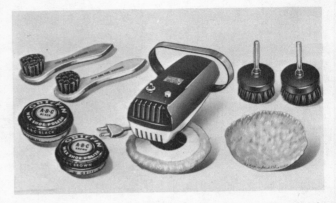

**FIG. 7-3.** Electric shoe-shiner with hand hold. The shiner's various attachments make it usable for other shining jobs also. (Courtesy of Sears Roebuck and Company, Chicago)

**FIG. 7-4.** A floor model electric shoe buffer. No hand work is required. (Sears Roebuck and Company, Chicago)

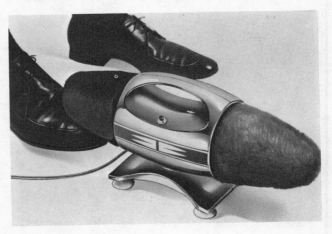

**FIG. 7-5.** Bath seat made from plastic wash basket (*A*). Child comfortably and safely seated for her bath (*B*). Her braces and shoes and socks will be removed when she bathes. (Courtesy of A. Slominski, Cerebal Palsy Clinic, Indiana University Medical Center)

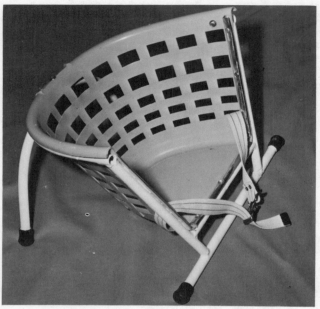

A

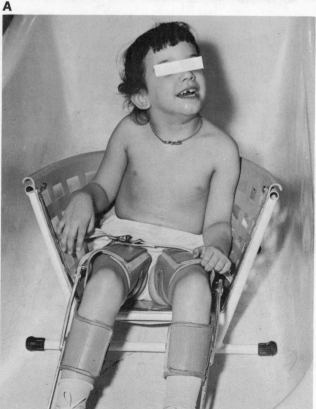

B

venience—many of them for self-help. Velcro tape has great versatility in the bathroom, holding various objects within easy reach of the user. A strip of pressure-sensitive Velcro hook tape applied to a wall near the sink can be used to hold a toothbrush, hand brush, or other toilet articles. Velcro pile tape is attached to the article to be held.

Consider, too, the use of shampoos that do not sting the eyes.

See the section on Mechanical Lifts in Chapter 3 for aids in getting a heavy or multiply handicapped person into and out of the bathtub or shower.

## SPECIAL TUB FOR A BABY

A small "life-size" plastic boat was purchased by the parents of a 2-year-old girl with cerebral palsy. They found it in a discount store for $8. Light enough for easy handling, the boat is placed on an old kitchen table in the basement and filled by hose from a faucet. The water is later siphoned off into the floor drain. The child is able to stretch out full length and paddle and splash to her heart's content. Bumps against the plastic sides cannot hurt, and the parents do not have to bend over to watch her and bathe her.

### Precautions

1. Make sure that any table on which such a tub is placed is large enough to provide a stable base so that the tub cannot tip off.
2. Place the tub on rubber mat or thin foam rubber padding to prevent slipping.

## TUB SEAT

A plastic wash basket has been used to make a clever bath seat (Fig. 7-5). One end is cut off, and a supporting frame made from electric conduit piping, welded and painted, holds the seat steady in the tub. A belt of webbing holds the child in place.

A chair with a seat approximately the same height as the side of the sub can also be used for an older child or adult. By grasping the bath rails, the bather can lower himself into the tub from the chair, which should be placed sideways to the tub (Fig. 7-6). Be sure, however, that the bather's hands and arms are strong enough for him to grasp the rails and to bear his weight.

## PORTABLE BATHING EQUIPMENT

Several items available at drugstores, general department stores, and catalog companies can make bathing safer and easier for teenagers and adults.

1. A rubber mat, with or without suction cups on the under side, to provide secure footing
2. Aluminum folding chairs with plastic webbing and rubber tips on the legs (crutch tips may fit)
3. Plastic-covered bath stools with aluminum legs and rubber tips
4. Portable shower hoses which can adjust to the tub faucet or to a nearby sink faucet if the hose is long enough
5. Portable shower hoses that slip over the head to hang around the neck. These are preferred by some individuals because they do not spray the hair and face.

Place a rubber mat in the tub and the chair or stool and adjust the shower hose. With such handy aids the patient can enjoy safe, seated bathing.

## SHOWER EXTENSION

A flexible shower extension, which will bring the nozzle to within easy reach of the seated bather, is available in many hardware stores or plumbing supply houses. It can be easily installed in place of the shower head. The flexible metal tubing makes it possible to raise the nozzle high where it will stay in place or to bring it down to any level convenient to the user. A loop of rubber tubing encircling the nozzle will protect against bumps.

**FIG. 7-6.** Chair at side of tub and special bathrails for older, stronger child. (Fro Svirsky, H. S. The severely involved child: Maternal backache. *Clin Orthop 47:*61, 1966. Reprinted with permission) (p. 48-Lipp.)

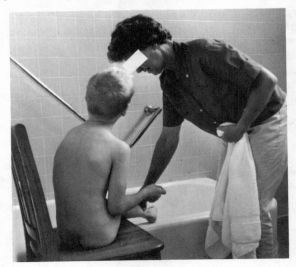

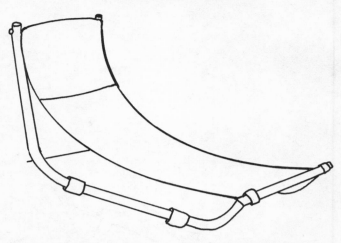

**FIG. 7-7.** Ideal Bathaide, made from nylon hammock on aluminum frame. (Courtesy of G. Crowder, Tucson, Ariz.)

## IDEAL BATHAIDE

The tub "recliner" is ideal for individuals with cerebral palsy (Fig. 7-7). The frame is constructed of noncorrosive aluminum tubing, reinforced by aluminum rods. The hammock is made of nylon, dries readily, and is strong. It has also been found useful in swimming pools and for sun bathing.

### Source

J. A. Preston Corp.
Sears Roebuck and Co., Medical Dept.

### Alternative

The aluminum chairs suggested under Portable Bathing Equipment, which come in sizes for adults or children, may also be used. A rubber mat should be placed in the tub and a portable shower hose used.

### BATH LIFT

A specially designed bath lift (Fig. 7-8) insures minimum effort for the person doing the lifting and maximum comfort for the patient. It is made of quick-drying, durable nylon webbing with dacron and comes in pink, white, blue, yellow, or wheat. Complete instructions for its proper use are included.

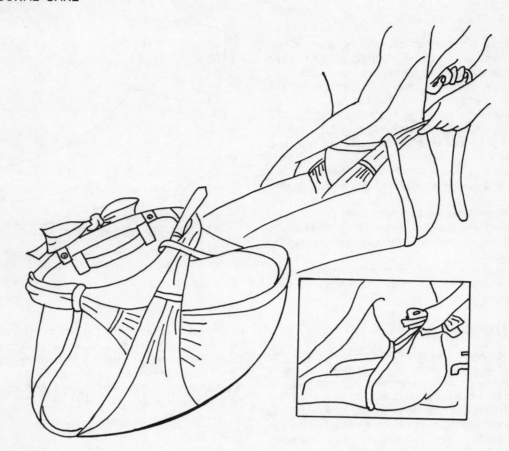

**FIG. 7-8.** Bath lift. Patient can be eased safely and comfortably into tub with little effort. (Courtesy of Vocational Guidance and Rehabilitation Services, Cleveland)

### Source

Vocational Guidance and Rehabilitation Services

### SOAP MITT

A self-help aid is a soap mitt (Fig. 7-9) made of terry cloth with two pockets (one for soap and one for the hand). It fastens around the wrist with Velcro and removes the problem of manipulating both soap and washcloth. It also eliminates the problem of soap that slips from the hand.

## ORAL HYGIENE AIDS

Maintenance of optimal oral hygiene often proves to be a complex problem for the physically handicapped. For example, because of breathing problems, some may have difficulty with any foaming type tooth paste. A dilute salt solution, made attractive by food coloring, is a useful substitute. The devices presented here have been developed by dentists and dental hygienists. The tooth and denture brushes were devised for use in a special project with the chronically ill and handicapped in Kansas City, Mo.

### Source for Dental Information

For information concerning dentistry for patients with cerebral palsy, write to:
Dental Guidance Council for Cerebral Palsy

### MASTI-CLEAN

An alternative to traditional brushing of the teeth is chewing on a spongy material, such as the Masti-Clean. The device is moistened and a small amount

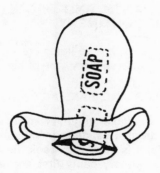

**FIG. 7-9.** Soap mitt made of terry cloth with Velcro wrist fastener. (Courtesy of United Cerebral Palsy of Denver)

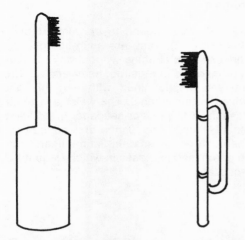

**FIG. 7-10.** Toothbrush for patient unable to grasp a smaller one (*A*), and one with elastic strap for patient unable to close his hands (*B*). (Courtesy of United Cerebral Palsy of Denver)

of dentifrice is applied. It is inserted into one side of the mouth and chewed up to 10 to 15 times. After the mouth is rinsed, the procedure is repeated on the other side of the mouth.

**Source**

Cleo Living Aids

## ROUND-HANDLED TOOTHBRUSH

For patients who are unable to grasp a regular toothbrush, a round-handled toothbrush may be helpful (Fig. 7-10*A*). It could be made out of clear plastic and spray-painted. Decals could also be used for decoration.

## TOOTHBRUSH WITH ELASTIC STRAP

An elastic strap secured onto the handle of a toothbrush (Fig. 7-10*B*) is especially suitable for patients who are unable to close their hands.

## ELECTRIC TOOTHBRUSHES

Some patients enjoy using electric toothbrushes, but it is advisable to check with the dentist first. Handles on electric toothbrushes differ, so try several to get the one with the most suitable grip. A handle with a flat surface does not roll when set down.

## NAIL BRUSH ADAPTED FOR CLEANING DENTURES

A nail brush with rubber suction cups attached will help a patient while he cleans dentures (Fig. 7-11*A*). The cups keep the brush in place on the sink, leaving the hands free to hold the dentures. An alternative is the nail brush with plastic handles which can be softened slightly and molded to fit the hand (Fig. 7-11*B*).

## MOUTHWASH

Mouthwash can be a problem for some patients to use without assistance. Put mouthwash into a plastic bottle and keep a plastic cup in the bathroom with a straw in it. A small amount of mouthwash can be poured into the cup from the bottle. With the aid of the straw, the patient can rinse his mouth with the mouthwash.

**FIG. 7-11.** Nail brushes adapted for cleaning dentures. (*Top*) Suction cups hold brush to sink, freeing hands. (*Bottom*) Handles have been molded to grip the hand. (Courtesy of United Cerebral Palsy of Denver)

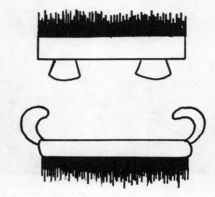

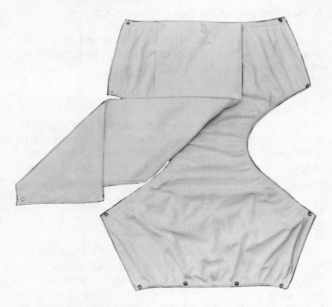

**FIG. 7-12.** Pro-Pants with a snap-in liner for protection of the incontinent. (Copyright 1965 by J. A. Preston Corporation)

**FIG. 7-13.** Sanitized Safe-T-Pants for protection of the incontinent. (Courtesy of Cleo Living Aids, Cleveland, Ohio)

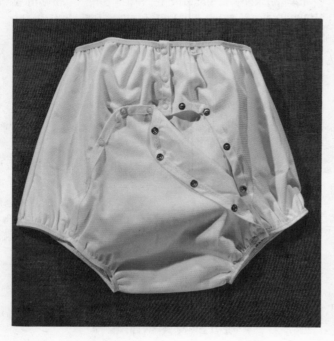

## SANITARY PANTS AND PROTECTION FOR THE INCONTINENT

A number of inexpensive items are available or can be made to facilitate sanitary care of the patient.

### PANTY SHIELDS AND SANITARY PANTS

These are available in junior miss and women's sizes at local drugstores, department stores, and catalog companies. It is helpful to hook the napkin to the belt or on the sanitary panty first and then have the wearer slip into them. Check whether the item is machine- or hand-washable before laundering.

### PRO-PANTS

Pro-Pants are designed to be comfortable as well as safe (Fig. 7-12). They are snug-fitting and can be worn under street clothing without any tell-tale bulge. They are made of thin-gauge, heat- and acid-resistant polyethylene plastic, lined with a highly absorbent Sanforized cotton flannel. The waist and thigh bands are elasticized to prevent seepage. In addition to the permanent lining, the pants are equipped with a detachable three-ply snap-in flannel liner. Extra liners can be purchased for cases in which frequent changes are necessary.

**Source**

J. A. Preston Corp.

### SAFE-T-PANTS

For patients with bladder or bowel difficulties, Safe-T-Pants afford maximum protection (Fig. 7-13). Made of rayon with waterproof coating, the pants are sanitized and have sealed-in protection that inhibits odor, germ growth, mildew, and rot.

**Source**

Cleo Living Aids
J. A. Preston Corp.

### SHOWER CAP URINAL

A plastic shower cap, beret style, can be made into a useful urinal for the "bed dribbler" during naps (Fig. 7-14). The shower cap should be seamless and stuffed with cellucotton. To keep the bed dry, the male patient may find it helpful to sleep on his abdomen with the shower cap placed under his genitalia.

A useful suggestion was made by readers of *Rehabilitation Gazette:* Bokon synthetic fibers placed firmly between the skin and any absorbent material will help to keep the skin dry. It is claimed that negative capillary action forces moisture through the Bokon, away from the skin. However, incontinence varies and a careful check should be made to remove these pads when they become moist near the skin. Bokon fibers are boilable, in contrast to Curity or Johnson & Johnson squares (24-inch or 36-inch squares) which are disposable.

## HOMEMADE SAFETY PANTS

This pattern (Fig. 7-15) will fit children size 10, weighing 83 lbs.
Materials: Muslin, broadcloth or other sturdy fabrics

**FIG. 7-14.** Urinal made from plastic shower cap lined with cellucotton. (Courtesy of New York University Medical Center, Institute of Rehabilitation, New York)

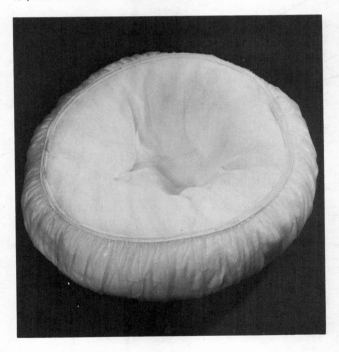

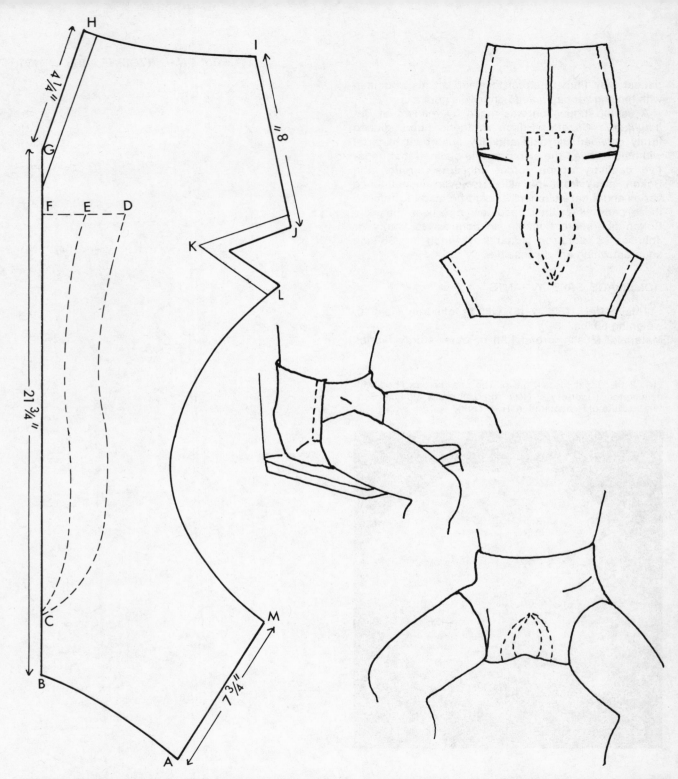

**FIG. 7-15.** Diagram for construction of home-made safety pants. *Left,* open pattern, showing position on fold of material. *Right, top,* open pants showing tape for closure; *center,* completed pants on patient; *bottom,* completed pants, front view, showing stitching lines of padding. (U. Haynes, United Cerebral Palsy, Inc., of New York)

that are washable and absorbent. Gripper tape, or velcro for closure.

Instructions:

1. Fold material lengthwise with points B, C, F, G, on fold. Points A, M and K are each 6 inches from fold. Cut two of pattern. Use left over scraps of fabric for padding in dotted areas C, D, E, F.
2. Sew darts GH and JKL.
3. Baste padding to one of the pieces of cut pattern, as indicated at CDEF.
4. With ¼ inch seam, join the two pieces of material cut to pattern, leaving a 4 inch opening for turning right side out.
5. Stitch padding, which has now been turned to the inside, firmly in place through both pieces of fabric.
6. Stitch 4 inch opening together.
7. Sew gripper or velco tape to each edge, AN and IJ, so as to ensure closure at sides with comfortable fit for leg openings.

Note: For male wearers, extra protection can be obtained by inserting the penis and scrotum into a plastic bowl cover or shower cap which has been stuffed with cotton. Be sure to extend thin layers of cotton over the edge of this container to prevent chafing.

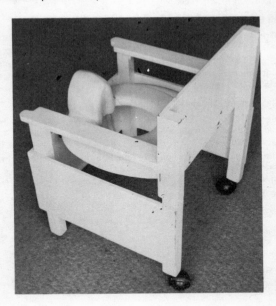

**FIG. 7-16.** A potty chair low enough for child's feet to rest on the floor. (From Svirsky, H. S. The Severely Involved Child: Maternal Backache. *Clin Orthop* 47:61, 1966. Reproduced with permission)

## TOILET AIDS FOR CHILDREN

Toilet training and care for children require that they be both comfortable and secure. If adaptations are not available, the child should be held while seated on the toilet so that he has no fear of falling. However, the greatest comfort and security are provided by a toilet or potty chair that is low enough for the child's feet to rest on the floor (Fig. 7-16) or on a footstool, and by some form of armrest and seat belt. A cut-out table going around the toilet allows the child's arms to rest and helps sitting balance. See section on Toilet Equipment in Chapter 1.

### MODIFIED TOILETS

For individuals with very little use of their hands, toilets can be installed which spray water for cleaning, eliminating use of toilet paper.

### Source

Sani-Seat, Inc.

# REFERENCES

### Safety in Bathtubs

Svirsky, H. S. "The severely involved child: Maternal backache," Clin Orthop 47:61, 1966.

### Oral Hygiene Aids

Greene, A. "A preventive guide for multi-handicapped children: Dental Care Begins at Home," Rehab Lit, 31:10–12, 1970.

Green, A., et al. "The electric toothbrush as an adjunct in maintaining oral hygiene in handicapped persons," J Dent Child 29:169, 1962.

### Toilet Aids for Children

Bensberg, G. J., ed. *Teaching the Mentally Retarded: A Handbook for Ward Personnel.* Atlanta, Southern Regional Education Board, 1966.

Brazelton, T. B. "A child-oriented approach to toilet training," Pediatrics 29:121, 1962.

Finnie, N. *Handling the Young Cerebral Palsied Child at Home.* New York, Dutton, 1970.

Kimbrell, D., Luckey, R., Barbuto, P., Love, J. "Operation dry pants for severely retarded: An intensive training program," Ment Retard 5:34, 1967.

Moore, P. "Toilet Habits Suggested for Training a Blind Child," American Foundation for the Blind.

Reaume, V. "Toilet Training as a Prerequisite for Admission to a Cerebral Palsy School," United Cerebral Palsy of Western New York.

Shriner, M. "Growing Up," National Easter Seal Society for Crippled Children and Adults.

### Professional Guides

ICTA Information Centre, Brooma, Sweden

"Self-Help Devices for the Handicapped: Bibliography," Library, National Easter Seal Society for Crippled Children and Adults.

Lawton, E. B. *Activities of Daily Living for Physical Rehabilitation.* New York, McGraw-Hill, 1963.

Lowman, E., Klinger, J. *Aids to Independent Living—Self-Help for the Handicapped.* New York, McGraw-Hill, 1967.

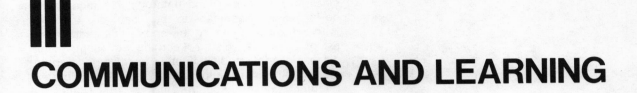

# III

# COMMUNICATIONS AND LEARNING

# 8
# Communication Aids

In this chapter and in Chapters 9 and 10, attention will be given to a variety of aids to learning for the handicapped. The emphasis will be upon the more informal aspects of education rather than upon formal schooling—what can be done in the home or care center, rather than in the schoolbuilding.

However, it is of paramount importance that the disabled youngster be able to attend school and to be physically functional within it. Stairs must not keep a child from his right to learn, and poorly designed classroom equipment and bathroom facilities should no longer add handicaps to the disabilities the child is trying to overcome. At the end of this chapter is a list of references on the Learning Environment that discuss needed modifications in buildings and equipment for the handicapped. See also the section and references on Architectural Barriers That Hinder the Physically Handicapped in Chapter 3.

Many of the aids discussed in this chapter are ones which can be used in the school environment as well as at home, and for the child who is able to attend school, it is advisable to discuss his needs with school personnel to be sure that home training will prepare him well and will suitably supplement his school work.

# SPEAKING SUBSTITUTES

## CONVERSATION BOARD

The conversation board offers a means of expression for those whose ability to do so in other ways is limited. Charts composed of useful words, signs, or numbers (Fig. 8-1) are covered with clear plastic and mounted securely on a desk of plywood board. The student uses his fingers or clenches a small dowel stick to point to letters, words, or numbers on the chart that he wishes to use. If he has no hand use, he may direct his eyes to words.

### Source for Information

The United Cerebral Palsy Association of New York State has a booklet, *Aphonic Communication for Those with Cerebral Palsy.* This is a guide for the development and use of a conversation board. Information on new findings developed since the publication of this booklet may be obtained from Miss Anne I. Remis of Rochester, N.Y.

### Precautions

1. Make the conversation board to fit the needs of the individual.
2. Start with a blank board and develop unit by unit, according to need.
3. Do not present any child who has not used the board before with a filled board.
4. Have separate boards for home use and for school use.

## MAGNETIC COMMUNICATION BOARD

A magnetic communication board can be obtained commercially or can be made. Letters of the alphabet, numbers, and "money" (Fig. 8-2) can be used on the board to learn to spell and count and then to communicate by building words.

**FIG. 8-1.** Conversation board. Child can communicate by pointing to words, numbers, or letters.

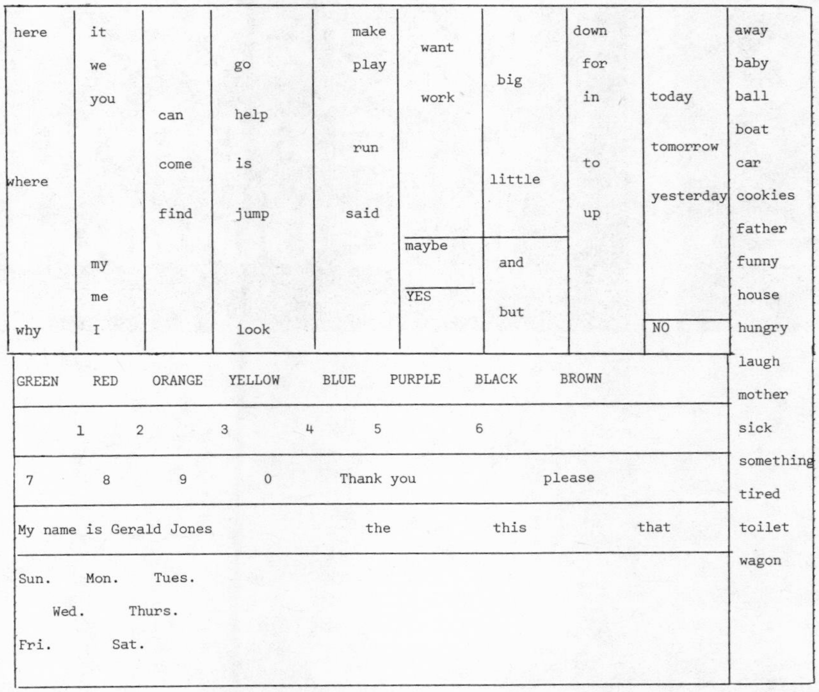

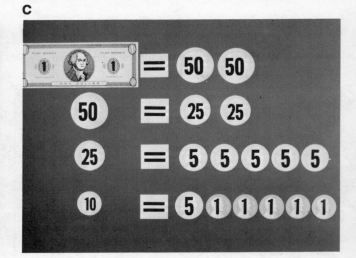

**FIG. 8-2.** Letters, numbers, and "coins" on a magnetic communication board. (Courtesy of Constructive Playthings. Kansas City, Mo.)

### Source

Constructive Playthings (Catalog available)

### Construction

Small magnets can be purchased at hardware or department stores. These can be attached by various methods such as gluing to toys, cardboard shapes, or other various items, or words cut from a page of large type. The items can then be placed on any piece of sheet metal or steel. Remember, aluminum will not hold magnets.

Magnets can also be placed along the edge of paper to hold it in place for crayoning or writing.

A table top or slant board covered with metal can make a useful surface for the child's play or school work. In housewares departments, look for magnets shaped like fruits and vegetables. These can be useful for counting, form and color recognition, as well as for securing paper and other objects.

### MECHANICAL COMMUNICATION BOARD

The Rick Communicator (Fig. 8-3), invented by Robert LaVoy, a teacher in San Mateo, Calif., has a panel with sufficient surface to display different types of information that the individual may want to convey to others. A pointer moves around the display panel to bring it into alignment with the information which the child wishes to convey.

The power to operate the pointer is controlled by an electric eye switch that can be attached to the child's desk or any other place suitable for him. The power can be initiated by a slight movement to break the beam of light. Finger, head, foot, or any part of the body that the child can control slightly will suffice. Once the beam of light is broken, the power means goes into effect and the pointer moves about the display panel.

When the child has the pointer aligned to the information, he removes the obstruction from the light and the pointer stops.

The father of one child adapted an electric switch to operate the panel in place of the electric eye. Such devices have been used successfully in teaching, reading, spelling, and number work. By this method a child can be tested on academic material presented to him, and he can be taught to make his basic wants known.

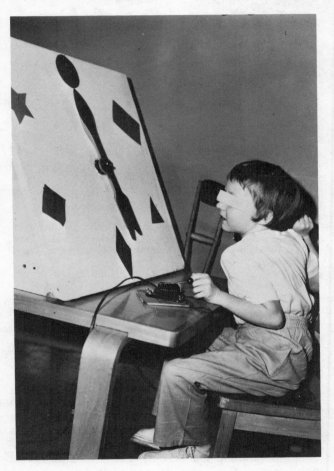

**FIG. 8-3.** The "Rick" mechanical communicator, adapted with an electrically driven pointer. By operating switch, child can move pointer to selected item. (From Jones, M. Electric communication devices. *Amer J Occup Ther 15:*110, 1961. Reproduced with permission)

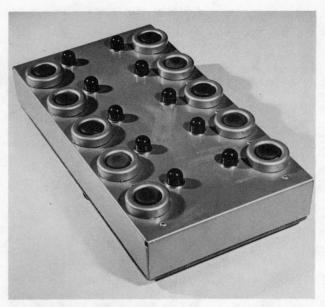

**FIG. 8-4.** Illuminaid. By pushing button, child can illuminate sign that conveys his message. (Courtesy of Bruce Wilson, Public Relations, Cleveland Electric Illuminating Co., Cleveland, Ohio)

United Cerebral Palsy Assn., San Mateo County, California.

ILLUMINAID

A device which can be made at home is the Illuminaid (Fig. 8-4), designed to help children who have no means of communication. It consists of a battery-run unit with 10 buttons that will turn on adjacent lights when pushed. Although the unit is compact, the buttons are carefully spaced and have protective raised rings around them that keep a child from pushing more than one at a time. Finger, toe, elbow, chin, etc., are among parts of the body that different children have used to operate Illuminaid.

Illuminaid can be used in a variety of ways, depending upon what sign is placed near each button. For example, simple instructions, such as "Drink, please," "Toilet, please," or "Yes" and "No," can cover many usual communications. For those who cannot read, pictures of needs may be used. On the other hand, signs can be made for numerals from 1 to 10 so that simple arithmetic can be learned. The adaptability of the unit depends upon the initiative of the adult who makes the signs useful to the needs and interests of the patient.

This device was developed for severely disabled youngsters at the Sunbeam School for Crippled Children in San Francisco by Bruce Wilson, Daniel Kovar, and Stanley Moskal of the Cleveland Electric Illuminating Company. All components of Illuminaid are standard parts available in any radio supply store, and the same store can even drill or punch the necessary holes in the chasis.

**Source for Manufacturing Instructions**

Instructions for construction are presented as a public service to help provide assistance to persons who have no means of communication. Write to: Bruce A. Wilson of the Cleveland Electric Illuminating Co.

# TYPEWRITERS

Typing is no longer confined to the strictly occupational uses by the general population or by the disabled. The only thing that cannot be translated from Cursive writing to a typewriter is an individual's signature. In our society, a typewriter is used for personal letters, homework, creative writing, schoolwork (Fig. 8-5), and other purposes on a wide scale. Robert Kendig writes in the *Cerebral Palsy Journal,* September 1965, that he uses a typewriter for postcards sent on vacations, for Christmas and birthday card messages, for mail-order shopping, accounts, checks, bills, pen pals, and even crossword puzzles!

For people with cerebral palsy who have speech disorders or severe arm and hand incoordination, typing is an essential means of communication. Typing for communication may be accomplished with one finger of one hand, one toe, or with some poking gadget attached to any part of the anatomy—forehead, chin, elbow, foot, or mouth. Anything that makes it possible for the disabled person to strike a typewriter key is a useful aid. Sometimes this can be accomplished on a regular typewriter by adjusting its height or position, placing it on the floor or on a firm pillow for footwork. Often a person can manage to press the keys of an electric typewriter, with or without a keyguard.

Sometimes remote control gadgets, developed experimentally all over the country, meet the individual's needs. These developments are reported from time to time in *Rehabilitation Gazette,* a publication specializing in information exchange between severely disabled individuals.

## SOURCES FOR USED ELECTRIC TYPEWRITERS

Used electric typewriters on an "as is" or reconditioned basis may be obtained at reduced rates from representatives of International Business Machines (IBM) in branch offices around the country. The IBM Branch Office Manual outlines a simple procedure which requires only that the purchase agreement be prepared bearing the following statement endorsed by a recognized organization interested in the welfare of handicapped persons or by a physician: "This purchase of an IBM electric typewriter is made for the use of a handicapped person." The manual also contains the following provision:

"Where it may present a problem for the handicapped person to obtain such an endorsement or the request for the endorsement may cause embarrassment unnecessarily, the Branch Manager may endorse the statement at his certification that the person is known to him and meets with the conditions of the order."

## PROS AND CONS FOR REVISED PLACEMENT

Revised placement of typewriter keys is controversial and should be done only upon consultation with an occupational therapist. It is possible to place the most used keys in a position on the keyboard that is more functional for some individuals. There is even a one-handed typewriter on the market. However, the user then becomes accustomed to exactly one machine, which may not be available in an employer's office, or the user may be left in a communication blackout during repair periods, which are inevitable with any mechanical apparatus.

## TYPEWRITER MODIFICATIONS AND TYPING AIDS

### KEYBOARD CHART

A heavy cardboard chart used in regular typing instruction has the letters and numerals of a typewriter keyboard enlarged and duplicated. A variation of this may be made of flannelboard, blackboard, or magnet board, depending on the teaching purposes. These charts may be placed flat or tilted for pointing with arms or pointers, or placed on the floor or on footstools for toe pointers. The objectives may be communication, spelling, or learning the keyboard via regular typing manual instructions.

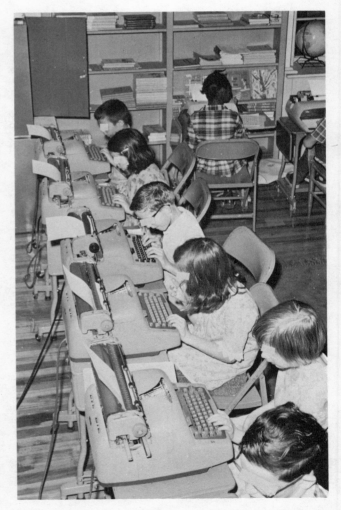

**FIG. 8-5.** Typewriter class for handicapped children. Typing can be a boon for those unable to write. (Courtesy of Spartanburg School for Handicapped Chidlren, Spartanburg, S.C.)

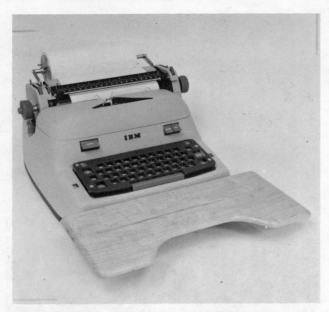

**FIG. 8-6.** Paper roll holder for typewriter. This machine also has an armrest and keyboard guard. The keyboard guard rests above keys, with a hole for each. When pointer is used to hit the keys, the guard helps to guide it. (Courtesy of International Business Machines)

**FIG. 8-7.** Diagram of table and armrest for typewriter. *A-B,* strap for arms; *C-D* and *E-G,* position of webbing for elbows or of back stop.

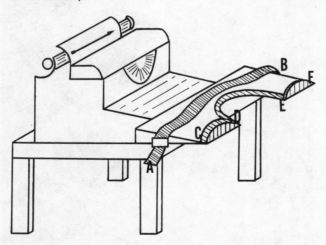

## PAPER ROLL HOLDER

A continual sheet of rolled paper 8 inches wide can be fed into a standard manual or electric typewriter from a paper roll holder (Fig. 8-6). The holder also has a built-in tear-off blade. The need to insert and remove individual sheets is thus eliminated.

### Source

International Business Machines, local branches

### TYPEWRITER TABLE AND ARMREST

A convenient typewriter table for the disabled person can be easily constructed (Fig. 8-7). It will help the typist control arm movement while seated comfortably at the machine.

### Construction

1. Cut off the legs of any sturdy table to the desired height for the typist.
2. Add an armrest built at the same angle as the keyboard of the typewriter. The armrest should have a cutout, within which the typist can sit and comfortably rest his arms up to the elbow.
3. Webbing strap or elastic (*AB*) will give the lower arms full horizontal sweep, while still helping to control them.
4. Some individuals may wish a web strap or wide elastic just below the elbow (*CD, EF*) for further security, or short padded backstops may be placed at these points to keep the elbows from sliding off the armrests.
5. The typewriter feet can be bolted to the table, if a rubber typing mat does not stabilize the machine in place.

### ONE-HANDED TYPING

It is possible for the person with the use of only one hand to learn to use the typewriter skillfully.

### Sources for Instruction

There are two publications which can help such an individual learn to type:

*Type with One Hand,* a book by Nina K. Richardson, published by Southwestern Publishing Company.

"A Method of Typing for the Handicapped: One-Hand Touch Typing," by LaVerna A. Smith, in *Cerebral Palsy Review,* November–December 1960, page 11.

## HEAD-POINTERS FOR NO-HAND TYPING

For persons unable to use their hands, several devices that can be purchased or made can help them learn to type.

1. A head band of elastic, tight enough to stay in place but not so tight as to cause a headache, can be made and a holder attached, into which a pointer can be inserted (Fig. 8-8). This one was designed by an occupational therapist at Oklahoma Cerebral Palsy Center in Norman. By nodding his head and aiming at the keys with the pointer, the typist is able to strike the key he selects. The device can be altered to suit the needs of the user.

2. A similar device is one with a cap, such as that used by H. Z., a student at University of California at Berkeley (Fig. 8-9). In the *Rehabilitation Gazette*, Mr. Z. writes:

   "The photograph shows my 'Woody Woodpecker' technique in typing. I use an IBM Selectric with perforated metal keyboard to prevent striking more than one key at a time. The helmet is hand-moulded to my skull with Elastoplast webbing glued into several layers by acetone application. To it is attached the dowel stick which I use for page turning when a removable pencil eraser is attached. I am strapped to a chair and my arms are 'handcuffed' at the wrists with webbing wristlets to control the 'overflow' motion caused by my athetoid cerebral palsy.

   "Thanks to the Selectric's various type-spheres, I am able to type Russian symbols and to make mathematical notations for college calculus."

3. A head-pointer that is adjustable in size and has a wand adjustable in length is available commercially (Fig. 8-10).

### Source

Fred Sammons, Inc.

## CHIN-POINTER FOR NO-HAND TYPING

A person who cannot talk may use a chin pointer (Fig. 8-11) to spell out words on a conversation board, as well as to type, write, paint, and play games. The chin piece is made of metal covered with a washable plastic, but some of the new moldable plastics or Fiberglas might also work. It is shaped to fit firmly around the chin and about halfway back on the jaw.

Straps, which snap in place on the chin piece, hold the piece to the head. A cross piece down the back joins the other two, creating a cap effect. A small

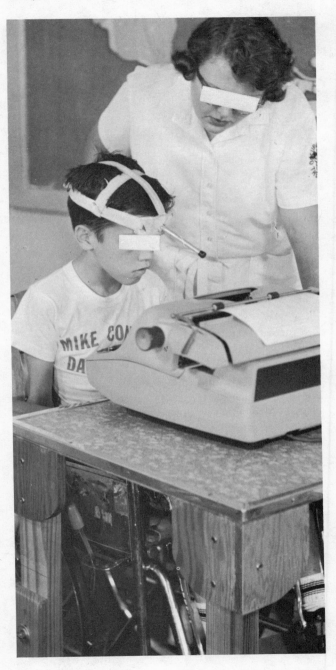

**FIG. 8-8.** Head-pointer on band, for no-hands typing. (Courtesy of Oklahoma Cerebral Palsy Center, Norman, Okla.)

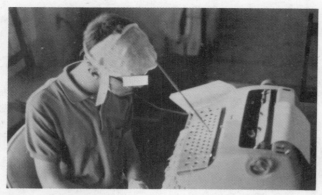

**FIG. 8-9.** Head pointer attached to hand-molded skull cap. (Courtesy of *Rehab Gaz.*, St. Louis, Mo.)

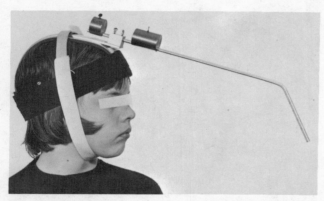

**FIG. 8-10.** Adjustable head-pointer, with head band and chin strap. (Courtesy of Fred Sammons, Inc., Brookfield, Ill.)

**FIG. 8-11.** Chin pointer for typing and other purposes. The young girl's arms were tied behind her back at her own request, since she discovered that her head control is better in this position. (Courtesy of E. Bell, Gonzalez Warm Springs Foundation, Tex.)

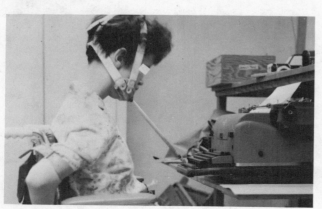

amount of elastic webbing in each of the straps helps to hold the apparatus firmly in place while allowing enough motion so that the wearer's chin does not feel completely bound down.

The pointer is a hollow metal tube into which a pointing stick can be inserted, or a pencil or paintbrush.

### VISTA

The Visual Instant Scanning Typewriter Adapter (VISTA) is designed for quadriplegics and persons with speech difficulties (Fig. 8-12). It is an electromechanical instrument for operating an electric typewriter. Only one movement is required to activate the switch, which can be depressed by any part of the body in which the user has controlled movement. When the machine begins to scan, the user again depresses the switch as soon as the correct letter lights up, and this in turn activates the key of the typewriter.

### Source

Bush Electric Company (The VISTA is used in connection with IBM Selectric 721 and other models.)

### MAGNETYPER

The Magnetyper was developed at the Rehabilitation Center of Hadley Memorial Hospital. It consists of an actuating box and a large composition panel board fitted with copper contacts the size of a silver dollar. The box sits over the keyboard of an electric typewriter. With a stylus attached to his head, the user can touch a letter on the control panel. This activates the box, from which a rod depresses the typewriter key.

### EXPERIMENTAL DEVICES

None of the aids described above are inexpensive, nor are any items that are made individually on an experimental basis. However, as research progresses and as items are made in larger quantities, they will eventually attain marketable prices. One, for example, is the Edison Responsive Environment Research Instrument (E.R.E. Machine) invented by Professor Omar K. Moore of Pittsburgh. This is being developed by the Thomas A. Edison Laboratory of West Orange, N.J., a division of the McGraw-Hill Company.

The Spring 1965 issue of *Rehabilitation Gazette*, contained reports of gadgets used by several multi-handicapped persons: a foot-operated coded type-writer; a "distaff" appliance; a gated, inertially matrixed control system; and an electronic multicontroller.

Dr. Suzanne Hill, Associate Professor of Psychology at Louisiana State University, is directing a project using electronic equipment to develop a program for teaching language skills to severely handicapped children. This project has received funds from the United Cerebral Palsy Research and Educational Foundation and the National Science Foundation.

## WRITING AIDS

### HOMEMADE PRACTICE AIDS

Several devices, easily and inexpensively contrived at home, can serve as practice aids for a handicapped person learning to write.

1. Cover a flat cookie baking tin with children's modeling clay. Use a stick or pencil to write in the clay.
2. Cover block oilcloth with white cleansing cold cream. Write with a finger.
3. Use finger paints on a washable surface.
4. Write with a wet sponge on a blackboard.
5. Melt old broken crayons. Pour into a cone-shaped paper drinking cup and let cool. When the wax is hard, fold the paper cup over the top and peel away the paper at the tip of the cup to expose the pointed end for coloring.

### MOUTHSTICK PENCIL HOLDER

A 14-inch wooden dowel with a mouthpiece shaped like that of a wind instrument is a useful device for the person without hand use (Fig. 8-13). The distal end is provided with a hole about $\frac{5}{16}$ inch wide and 1½ inches deep, into which a pencil, paintbrush, or pointer can be inserted. The center area of the stick can be sanded down to about ⅜ inch to lighten its weight. The stick could also be made out of a plastic or nylon.

### DOWELING PENCIL HOLDER

A hole drilled through a piece of dowel will make a satisfactory pencil holder (Fig. 8-14). A screw into the end of the dowel will keep the pencil from slipping. The eraser end of the pencil can be used to tap the keys of a typewriter.

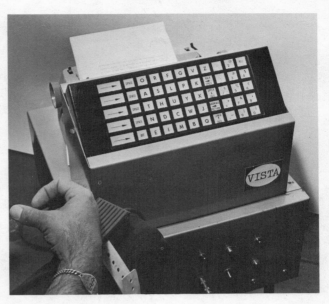

**FIG. 8-12.** Visual Instant Scanning Typewriter Adapter. Switch can be depressed by any controlled part of the body. (Courtesy of Bush Electric Co., San Francisco, Calif.)

**FIG. 8-13.** Mouthstick for typing and other purposes, made from wooden dowel with shaped mouthpiece. (Courtesy of UCPA, Inc.)

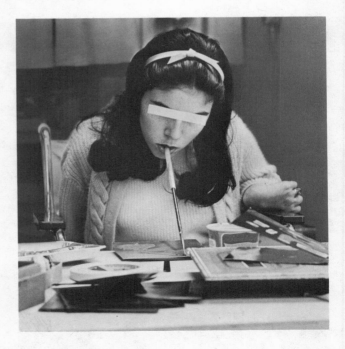

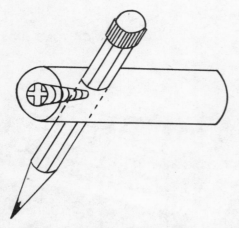

**FIG. 8-14.** Diagram of wooden dowel used as pencil holder.

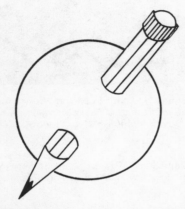

**FIG. 8-15.** Sponge rubber ball used as pencil holder.

**FIG. 8-16.** Sarong pencil holder, with Velcro wrap for the fingers. (Courtesy of Fred Sammons, Inc., Brookfield, Ill.)

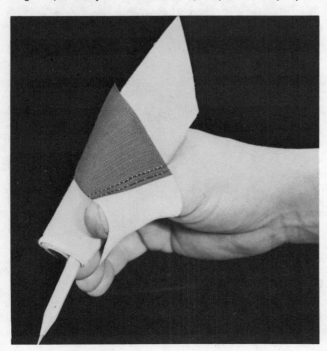

## SPONGE BALL PENCIL HOLDER

A pencil pushed through a sponge rubber ball is also useful (Fig. 8-15). This too can be used for typing purposes.

## SARONG PENCIL HOLDER

A commercially available holder is made of Velcro (Fig. 8-16). The tape encapsulates the pencil, then wraps around the fingers and thumb to hold the pencil at the correct writing angle. It will not slip off, yet is comfortable over long periods of time. It comes in a pleasant beige and brown combination.

### Source

Fred Sammons, Inc.

## SIDE-WINDER PENCIL HOLDER

Fastened to the hand by a band, this utensil holder provides writing function without grasp (Fig. 8-17). A locking mechanism holds the pencil firmly in place. It comes in stainless steel, and is for the right hand.

### Source

Fred Sammons, Inc.

# READING AIDS

## MOUTHSTICK PAGE TURNER

A handy mouthstick for turning the pages of a book is specially designed to help prevent damage to the teeth, which can occur following long-term use of such a stick (Fig. 8-18). The mouthpiece of a snorkel tube is applied to one end of a light-weight, thin aluminum tube. A suction cap attached to the other end grasps the page. See similar devices in C. Rosenberg, *Assistive Devices for the Handicapped.* Minneapolis, American Rehabilitation Foundation, 1968.

Vinyl, arcylic, and liquid latex have also been used for the mouthpieces on mouthsticks.

## MAGNETIC MOUTHSTICK PAGE TURNER

Instead of a suction cup, a small cylindrical magnet can be used. On this stick, devised at the Self-Help Device Workshop at the New York University

Medical Center, Institute of Rehabilitation Medicine, the magnet is attached with Scotch tape or a fiber sleeve. Paper clips are placed on each page of the book to be read, and the magnet lifts the page when it touches the clip.

## DOWEL AND MAGNET PAGE TURNER ON HEADBAND

A simple page turner on a headband can be easily made (Fig. 8-19). It consists of an aluminum band, fastened to the head with elastic. A dowel attached to the band has a magnet page turner on the end. Paper clips or other small metal pieces are attached to each page near the outside center. Very useful for this purpose are the metal clips with colored tabs that are used on file cards. As the magnet contacts the metal clip, the page is picked up; the user then completes the operation by a right-to-left motion of the head.

### Construction

1. Cut a band (A) of thin aluminum 2 inches wide and 12 inches long (Fig. 8-20).
2. Bend the band to a "U" shape, and drill a hole at each end (B).
3. Attach a wooden dowel (C), ½ inch in diameter and 6 inches long to the band by a small screw. The screwhole (D) must be countersunk to make the screw level with the inside surface of the band.
4. To the other end of the dowel, attach the magnet (E) by a screw soldered to the magnet.
5. Pull a double strip of elastic through the holes (B) in the headband to hold it securely. The inner surface of the band can be lined with ¼-inch sponge rubber for greater comfort. A piece of stockinette sewed around the band covers the sponge rubber and provides friction so that the band stays in place on the forehead.

### Precaution

If the stick is adapted for writing or painting, check with an eye doctor for visual field and focal point of each wearer.

## WAND AND SUCTION CUP PAGE TURNER ON HEADBAND

A suction cup can be attached to a plastic straw, which can then be slipped onto a head wand and fastened (Fig. 8-21). See similar devices in C. Rosen-

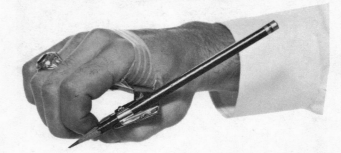

FIG. 8-17. Side-winder pencil holder, with locking mechanism to grip pencil tightly. (Fred Sammons, Inc., Brookfield, Ill.)

FIG. 8-18. Page turner with snorkel mouth piece. (Courtesy of C. Rosenberg)

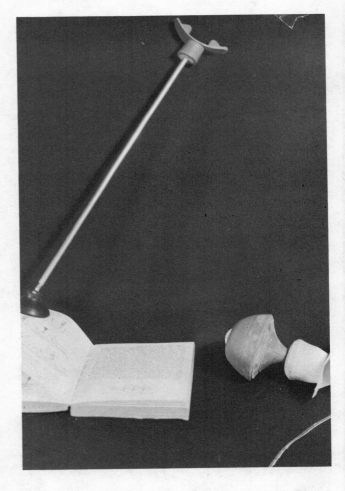

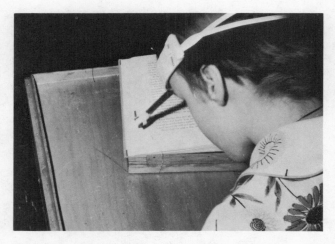

FIG. 8-19. Head-band page turner with magnets to contact metal clips on pages. (From Lauretana, M., and Liepmann, D. Head-band page turner. *Amer J Occup Ther 11:*75, 1957. Reproduced with permission)

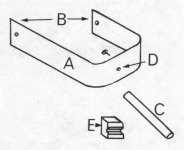

FIG. 8-20. Diagram for construction of page turner with magnets. *A,* aluminum band; *B,* holes for elastic; *C,* dowel stick; *D,* hole to screw dowel to band; *E,* magnet. (From Lauretana, M., and Liepmann, D. Head-band page turner. *Amer J Occup Ther 11:*75, 1957. Reproduced with permission)

FIG. 8-21. Page turner with suction cup attached to plastic straw in a head wand. (Courtesy C. Rosenberg, *Assistive Devices for the Handicapped* Minneapolis, Am. Rehab. Foundation, 1968, Reproduced with permission)

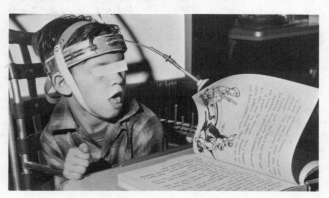

berg, *Assistive Devices for the Handicapped.* Minneapolis, American Rehabilitation Foundation, 1968.

## BALL AND SUCTION CUP PAGE TURNER FOR HAND USE

The patient with some ability to grasp can use a sponge rubber ball to which a suction cup or half a hollow rubber ball is attached (Fig. 8-22). See similar devices in C. Rosenberg, *Assisting Devices for the Handicapped.* Minneapolis, American Rehabilitation Foundation, 1968.

## WASHER ATTACHED TO BAND USED AS PAGE TURNER

A soft rubber washer attached to a band that straps to the wrist or elbow could be used for the patient with poor hand use. Or a metal washer that has been magnetized could be sewed to a band and used to contact paper clips or metal tabs on the page.

## LAKELAND AUTOMATIC PAGE TURNER PC 7602

This page turner accepts the largest and smallest magazines, hardback books and paperback books. It can be easily and quickly set up, and once the book or magazine is in place, the operation is very simple. Only a momentary light touch (movement of less than ¼ inch) by any part of the body is necessary to operate the sensitive control switch. A silicone-coated arm picks up the page and turns it; a second arm holds the turned pages in place.

The page turner is of all metal construction with overall dimensions of 14 by 24 inches, and is finished in soft green with nickel-plated parts. It weighs only 12½ pounds and is easily placed on any overbed table, work table, or wheelchair tray. Standard units operate on a 110- to 120-volt, 50- to 60-cycle outlet. Instructions for use are provided.

**Source**

J. A. Preston Corp.

## TURN-A-PAGE PC 7605

Another automatic page turner that accommodates all sizes from large magazines down to small books has microswitches to turn the pages forward or backward. The switches require only a slight touch and may be placed next to the patient wherever he can exercise movement. The Turn-A-Page measures 24 by 20 inches, and can be placed on the patient's lap, on a bed table, or on a wheelchair tray.

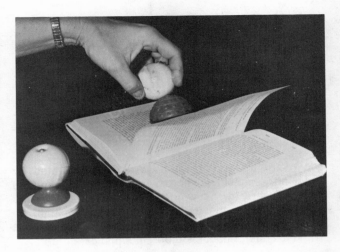

**FIG. 8-22.** Sponge ball attached to half a rubber ball for page turner. Sponge ball can also be attached to suction cup (*lower left.*) (Courtesy C. Rosenberg. American Rehabilitation Foundation, 1968. Reproduced with permission)

## Source

J. A. Preston Corp.

## Precautions

Consult the nearest chronic disease hospital or rehabilitation center to determine the advantages and disadvantages of the different models of automatic page turners for the different stresses placed upon them. Also discuss the amount of use given the machine. Investigate the amount of help needed to set up each machine, the repair contracts, and whether repairs can be done locally.

## TALKING BOOKS

A wide variety of talking books and magazines is now available for handicapped persons from several sources.

In 1966 the Library of Congress was authorized to extend its national program of Books-for-the-Blind to residents of the United States and to U.S. citizens abroad who cannot read conventional printed materials because of physical limitations.

Readers with these handicaps may now borrow talking books through 34 cooperating regional libraries in the United States that already serve blind readers. The service is entirely free.

To borrow books from one of the regional libraries, the applicant should obtain from a competent authority a brief statement certifying the characteristics of his physical disability. The statement should come from a doctor, optometrist, registered nurse, profes-

sional staff member of a hospital or other institution or agency, or, in the absence of any of these, from a professional librarian. In cases of total blindness, a statement signed by a prominent member of the community is accepted. The statement should be sent to the regional library for the blind in the person's area or, if he does not know its identity, to the Library of Congress.

More than two dozen phonographs and record sets have already been obtained for children and adults with cerebral palsy in New York State through the affiliates and United Cerebral Palsy Association of New York State.

The books are general in scope, ranging from titles of current and popular interest to classics and vocational and practical materials. Also available are several well-known magazines, such as *American Heritage, Holiday, Good Housekeeping,* and *Sports Illustrated.*

*Talking Book Topics,* a bimonthly review of the new talking books produced for the Library of Congress, is available for loan through various distributing libraries.

### Sources

Division for the Blind and Physically Handicapped, Library of Congress, Washington, D.C. 20542 (catalogs of books available in the regional libraries and information on national services and resources)

American Foundation for the Blind. (publisher of *Talking Book Topics*)

Complete catalogs are available from:

Audio Book Co.
Caedmon Records Inc.
Enrichment Records
Folkway Records
Curtis Circulation Co., School Division
Spoken Arts, Incorporated
Swann. Borrow from your record store

### FILMED BOOKS

Projectors are available for showing enlargements of filmed books. One casts the enlargement on the ceiling; movement is controlled by light pressure. About 1,300 books are available. Another compact, light-weight projector can cast the image overhead, or on a wall or screen. It is suitable for small rooms and operates on 110 to 112 volts AC with a 400-watt lamp.

### Sources

3M Company, Visual Products

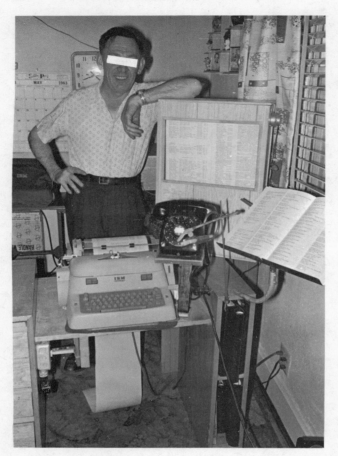

**FIG. 8-23.** Roll-o-Matic, for information storage. Microswitch to operate device can be adapted for handicapped user. (Courtesy of C. Park, Lima, Ohio and *Rehab Gaz;* St. Louis, Mo.)

**FIG. 8-24.** Amplifier and speaker for telephone to aid handicapped user. (Courtesy of Heritage House, Wallingford, Pa.)

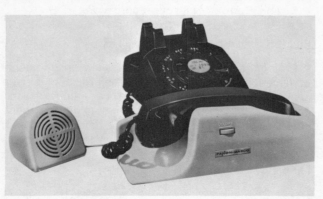

### ROLL-O-MATIC

A gadget for information storage, the Roll-O-Matic is a flat wooden box with a window opening (Fig. 8-23). It holds a continuous paper roll, about 4 feet long and 15 inches wide. On this roll, the user can list addresses, telephone numbers, birthdays, membership rosters, price lists, schedules, tables—anything at all that one might wish to have handy for frequent use.

The paper rolls in one direction, upward. The electric motor that operates the device is activated by pressing a sensitive microswitch. When the needed data appears in the window, the switch is pressed again to stop the roll. The microswitch can be mounted in various ways to allow the user to touch it with his finger, head, shoulder, mouthstick, or foot.

**Source**

Charles Park

## TELEPHONE MODIFICATIONS

Several modifications of the standard telephone handset are available, most of them designed to meet a specific problem of the handicapped person. The user's ability to use his hand or some other part of the anatomy to turn switches on and off or to lift the handset should be considered in making a selection.

Your local Bell System (AT&T) educational specialist can discuss how schools can use computer-assisted instructions and how TeleClass can keep the home-bound person in communication with his class.

### 3-A SPEAKERPHONE

The 3-A Speakerphone, made by American Telephone and Telegraph Company, has a microphone and loudspeaker attached to the desk phone. This lets the user talk and listen without touching the regular handset.

**Source**

Local telephone company

### AMPLIFIER FOR TELEPHONE

This aid allows the user to lay the telephone receiver on a cradle of the amplifier (Fig. 8-24). The weight of the receiver pushes down a button on the cradle, which turns on the amplifier. He can then hear as well as answer from a distance of up to 6 feet.

## Source

Heritage House

## DIALING MOUTHSTICK

To enable a person with poor hand use to dial a telephone, Imogene Prichard, a reader of *Rehabilitation Gazette,* suggests the use of a mouthstick. It is made of a 7-inch length of nylon and has one end flattened and grooved to allow the user to get a secure grip with his jaw teeth. Actually the pushbutton type of handset makes dialing easier for hands or mouthstick.

## AUTOMATED CARD DIALER

Frequently used numbers can be coded on plastic cards for use with the Card Dialer phone (Fig. 8-25). The desired card is pushed into a slot. The user then lifts the hand set, waits for the dial tone, presses the "start" bar and waits for an answer. The cards are filed alphabetically right in the telephone box, where they are always handy.

## Source

Local telephone company

## MAGICALL

The Magicall contains telephone numbers frequently used by the owner. They are stored on magnetic tape and are visibly indexed. Only the ability to press a button to start and stop the mechanism is needed.

## Source

Local telephone company

## SENSICALL

A Sensicall set helps the deaf, the deaf-blind, or the mute to use the telephone via the International Morse Code (Fig. 8-26). Model TN-9 enables the user to employ voice signals or push-button signals which the Sensicall converts into short or long flashes of light.

Model TB-9 enables the blind user to receive messages by a sense of touch by placing the finger or a button that converts the Morse Code into vertical motions.

## Source

American Telephone & Telegraph Company

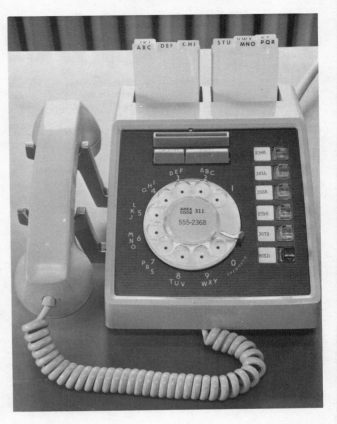

**FIG. 8-25.** Card dialer telephone for frequently used numbers. (Courtesy of American Telephone and Telegraph Company, New York)

**FIG. 8-26.** Sensicall set, by which user can employ Morse code signals for telephoning. (Courtesy of American Telephone and Telegraph Company, New York)

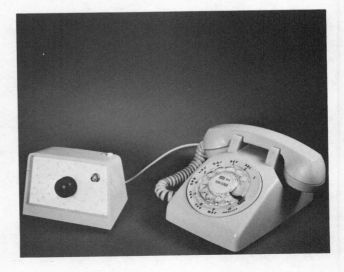

# REFERENCES

**The Learning Environment**

"American Standards Association Specifications for Making Buildings and Facilities Accessible to, and Usable by, the Physically Handicapped," National Easter Seal Society for Crippled Children and Adults, Inc., 1961.

"Architectural Workshop: Conference Report of Artichitectural Institute" Portland, Oregon, National Association for Retarded Children, 1967.

"Design for All Americans," Superintendent of Documents, U.S. Government Printing Office, Washington, D.C. (50 cents)

*The Design of a Pre-school "Learning Laboratory" in a Rehabilitation Center,* New York, New York University Medical Center, Institute of Rehabilitation Medicine, 1969.

*Making Facilities Accessible to the Physically Handicapped,* Albany, State University Construction Fund, 1969.

*Modification of Educational Equipment and Curriculum for Maximum Utilization by Physically Disabled Persons:* No. 8, Yuker, H., Revenson, J. and Fraschia, J.—"Design of a School for Physically Disabled Students," 1968; No. 9, Yuker, H., Feldman, M., Fraschia, J., and Young, J.,—"Educational and School Equipment by Physically Disabled Students," 1967; No. 12, Nemarich, S. and Velleman, R.,—"Curriculum and Instructional Techniques," 1969. Human Resources Center, Albertson, New York

Schoenbaum, W. *Planning and Operating Facilities for Crippled Children,* Springfield, Ill., Charles C Thomas, 1962.

"Housing for Early Childhood Education," Bulletin 22-A, Association for Childhood Education, Internationak, 1968.

**Keyboard Chart**

"Teaching Aids for Children with Cerebral Palsy," New York State Education Department, Bureau of Physically Handicapped Children, 1966.

**Mechanical Communication Board**

Jones, M. "Electrical communication devices," Amer J Occup Ther 15:110, 1961.

**Magnetyper**

Evans, A. J. "Meet the Magne-typer, J Rehab 26:32, 1960.

**Mouthsticks**

Buckley, R., Slominski, A. "Acrylic mouthpiece, Am J Occup Ther 12: 23–25, 1958.

Prichard, I. Rehabilitation Gazette 24, Spring 1964.

Thorpe, S., Wells, R. "Liquid latex mouthpiece," Am J Occup Ther 11:73–74, 1957.

Yeakel, M. "Vinyl Mouthpiece," Biomechanical Research Laboratory, Walter Reed Army Hospital.

Lauretana, M., Liepmann, D. "Head-band page turner," Am J Occup Ther 11:75, 1957.

Rosenberg, C. *Assistive Devices for the Handicapped,* Minneapolis, American Rehabilitation Foundation.

Sullivan, R. A., Frieden, F. H., Cordery, J., "Telephone Services for the Handicapped," New York University Medical Center, Institute of Rehabilitation Medicine.

# 9
# Learning Aids for Children

Learning opportunities and professional guidance for both parents and children during a child's infancy and preschool years are essential to rehabilitation. This chapter will present a number of learning aids for children during this period and during early school years. The selection has been made with the particular needs of the handicapped child in mind and emphasizes fun and formative experiences.

### Sources for Information

A practical overview of educational planning for children with cerebral palsy is *Realistic Educational Planning for Children with Cerebral Palsy. Preschool Years,* published by United Cerebral Palsy Associations, Inc.

Another helpful source is *Adapting Materials for Educating Blind Children with Sighted,* published by New York State Education Department, Bureau for Physically Handicapped Children.

## AIDS TO DEVELOPING CONCEPTIONS OF SPACE, SIZE, COLOR, AND SHAPE

Toys that are designed with the twofold purpose of play and learning best serve any child's needs (Fig. 9-1). Consult toy and school catalogs and then make the adaptations needed for informal and planned learning opportunities.

### SOURCES FOR MATERIALS AND INFORMATION

For manipulative materials that require simple to complex skills, write for catalogs to:

Childcraft Education Corp. (*Childcraft . . . Toys That Teach*)

Community Playthings

Constructive Playthings

Creative Playthings (*Aids to Learning; A Child's Way of Learning; Equipment Checklist; A Headstart for Every Child*)

General Learning Corp. (The Judy Co.) (Visual Manipulative Materials)

Kenner Products

J. A. Preston Corp. (Catalog 1080, Supplement A)

**FIG. 9-1.** Toys as learning aids. Children begin to develop concepts of size, color, and shape by handling toys. (Courtesy of Children's Hospital School, Eugene, Ore.)

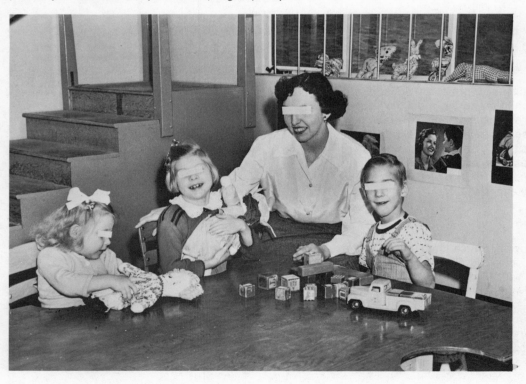

For teaching aids that may be three-dimensional, magnetic, or visuotactile, write for catalogs issued by:

Appleton-Century-Crofts
Book-Lab, Inc.
Developmental Learning Materials Inc.
EduKaid of Ridgewood
The Continental Press, Inc.
Ideal School Supply Co.
R. H. Stone Products

## AIDS TO PERCEPT AND CONCEPT DEVELOPMENT

Montessori materials offer a wide range of graded sensorial experience. A child can select activities which start at his individual level of success and get feedback from progressive stages. In this sense the materials offer self-corrective, play-learning opportunities.

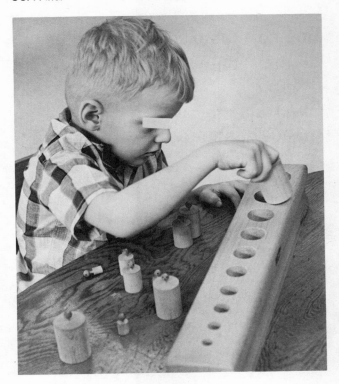

**FIG. 9-2.** Montessori size box. Child not only learns to relate sizes but begins to develop some dexterity. (Courtesy of United Cerebral Palsy of New Orleans) 1967 Annual Rep. UCPA Inc.

For materials and information related to Montessori methods (Fig. 9-2) write to:

*Children's House Magazine,* Inc.
Educational Teaching Aids (Teaching Aids Catalog)

Frostig materials and techniques offer two- and three-dimensional experiences within six areas of a child's physical and mental growth. As defined by Marianne Frostig these six areas are: Motor, perceptual, intellectual, emotional and social development, plue language.

For a descriptive outline of Frostig materials, write to:

Follett Publishing Co.
Marianne Frostig Center of Educational Therapy

For materials published especially for parents and professionals teaching children who are slow learners or have learning disabilities, and for teachers of all children in the preschool and lower grades, write to:

Teaching Resources

Associates serving Teaching Resources in its evaluation and product development are: William Cruickshank, Ph.D., Jean R. Hebeler, Ed.D., Belle Dubnoff, M.A., and Elizabeth S. Freidus, M.A. The materials presently available are: Ruth Cheves Program of Visual-Motor Perception Teaching Materials; Erie Program of Perceptual-Motor Teaching Materials; Fairbanks-Robinson Program of Perceptual-Motor Development; Dubnoff School Program of Sequential Perceptual-Motor Exercises; and Pathway School Program of Eye-Hand Coordination Exercises.

For information concerning specialized perceptual training activities for application in the classroom, write to:

Teachers College Press

Particularly helpful is the *Perceptual Training Activities Handbook,* by Betty Van Witsen. This is part of the Teachers College Series in Special Education. It illustrates that perception can be taught through the provision of planned sensory experience and interpretation in vision, language, gesture, kinesthesis, and touch. Frances Connor, Ph.D., is editor of the series.

### TYPEWRITER GAMES

Tapping on a typewriter can be fun and help to develop coordination and to teach letters and spelling (Fig. 9-3). The preschooler can set a toy car on top of the type roller and make it move from left to right by depressing the space bar. He can be taught to put it back for another ride by using the carriage return handle. He can also be taught to match letters, using the hunt-and-peck system.

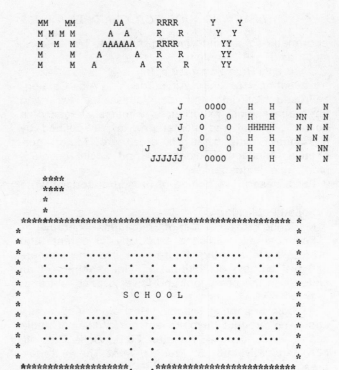

```
  MM   MM      AA     RRRR     Y   Y
  M M M M     A  A    R   R     Y Y
  M  M  M    AAAAAA   RRRR       YY
  M     M    A    A   R   R      YY
  M     M    A    A   R   R      YY


            J    0000   H   H    N    N
            J   0    0  H   H    NN   N
            J   0    0  HHHHH    N N  N
            J   0    0  H   H    N  N N
        J   J   0    0  H   H    N   NN
        JJJJJJ   0000   H   H    N    N


    ****
    ****
     *
     *
  ***********************************************  *
  *                                                *
  *                                                *
  *    .....   .....   .....   .....   .....  ....  *
  *    .   .   .   .   .   .   .   .   .       .  . *
  *    .   .   .   .   .   .   .   .   .....   .  . *
  *                 S C H O O L                    *
  *    .   .   .   .   .   .   .   .   .   .   .    *
  *    .   .   .   .   .   .   .   .   .   .   .    *
  *    .....   .....   .   .   .....   .....   .... *
  *               .   .       .                    *
  *                 .       .                       *
  ***********************. . .********************
```

**FIG. 9-3.** Typewriter games. Learning to make pictures with a typewriter helps develop coordination and learn letters and spelling.

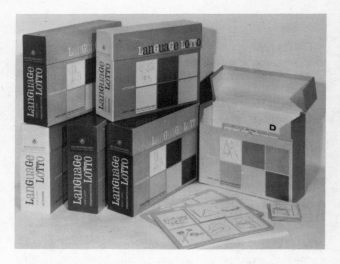

**FIG. 9-4.** Language Lotto. Game helps children to learn English. (Courtesy of Appleton-Century-Crofts, New York)

As the child grows older, he can learn to type words or make pictures with the hunt-and-peck system (Fig. 9-3), using a finger or fingers, or any part of the body. In fact, with a child who has poor hand use, all parts of the body can be tried to find which method can be used with the greatest ease.

## AIDS TO LANGUAGE DEVELOPMENT

There are several fine sources which can be used to help the child to develop a good vocabulary.

### LANGUAGE LOTTO GAME

This is a series of programmed games to teach children to understand and to speak standard English (Fig. 9-4). A teacher's guide is provided with the washable card sets.

**Source**

Appleton-Century Crofts

### PEABODY LANGUAGE DEVELOPMENT KITS

Lessons and materials in this system are designed to stimulate overall language development (Figs. 9-5 and 9-6). The lessons are divided into two levels: Level 1 for mental age 4½ to 6½ and Level 2 for mental age 6 to 8. The materials include: a manual for the teacher; 2 puppets; color cards; tapes; plastic color

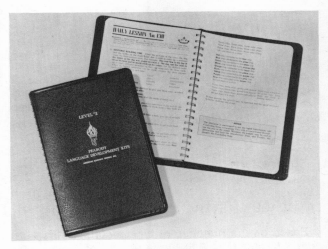

**FIG. 9-5.** Manual for Peabody language development kit. (Courtesy of American Guidance Service, Inc., Circle Pines, Minn.)

chips; wonder posters; and a teletalk intercom system.

### Source

American Guidance Service, Inc.

## PERIODICALS

Parents will find helpful suggestions in several journals related to child development.

### Sources

Children Today (formerly *Children*)
*Children's House Magazine*
*Today's Child*

## TAPE RECORDER

The tape recorder is a valuable teaching aid as it may be used with individuals or with groups and the material can be prepared in advance, allowing the teacher more time for other pupils. The volume of work can be adjusted to needs and abilities. The tape recorder has been helpful in promoting attention span, in recording scripts to be used with puppets in learning situations, and in learning from playbacks at group counseling sessions.

Multiple outlets with individual earphones may be attached to any tape recorder's external speaker.

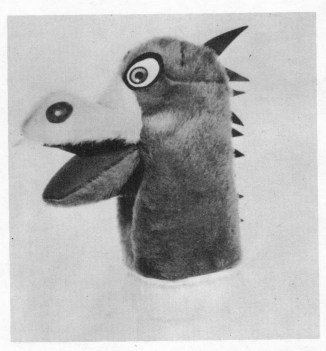

**FIG. 9-6.** Puppet from Peabody language development kit. (Courtesy of American Guidance Service, Inc., Circle Pines, Minn.)

## MOBILE LEARNING CENTER

The Mobile Learning Center (Fig. 9-7) has a capacity for eight persons. The set includes tape, a phonograph, and external input attachments. All that needs to be added is the teacher's voice. It can also be used for the individual child.

**Source**

American Seating Co.

## LANGUAGE MASTER

Based on the principle of tape recording, the Language Master (Fig. 9-8) has a variety of material for individual and group use. As the card is inserted, the child sees the picture and the printed word and hears the word pronounced. Among the materials available are those on vocabulary, world learning, language stimulation, English development, sounds of English, and phonics.

**FIG. 9-7.** Mobile Learning Center. Equipment can be used by a group or by an individual. (Courtesy of American Seating Co., Grand Rapids, Mich.)

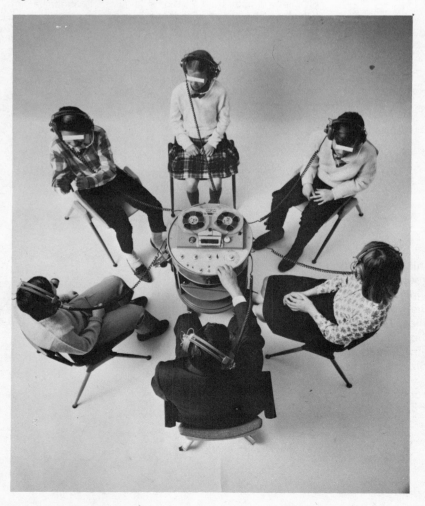

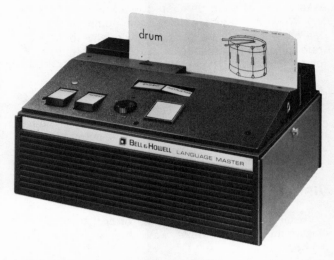

**FIG. 9-8.** Language Master for individual or group use. Printed word and picture are shown as word is spoken. (Courtesy of Bell & Howell, Chicago)

**Source**

Bell & Howell Co.

## AIDS FOR LEARNING NUMBERS AND ARITHMETIC

Learning numbers and simple arithmetic can be fun because so many games make use of numbers.

### TEN GIANT STEPS TO RECOGNITION

This "pathway" to learning numbers was designed by Candice Latham, a teacher at Eldredge Park School, Binghamton, N.Y. On a board or mat, ten footprints are painted (Fig. 9-9). Each print contains a number from 1 to 10 and dots adding up to the number printed. This board could serve a dual purpose for the disabled child learning to walk, since he can practice walking while he learns to count.

### ARITHMETIC BOARD

Another handy aid, also devised by Miss Latham, is the arithmetic board, which can be easily made. At one edge of the board are printed the numbers 1 to 10, each in a separate block. Attached to the board by

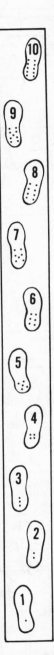

**FIG. 9-9.** Diagram of chart for 10 Giant Steps to Recognition. Child can make a game of learning numbers and counting. (From Latham, C. *Teaching Aids for Children with CP.* Albany, N.Y., Bureau for Physically Handicapped Children. Reproduced with permission)

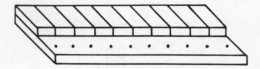

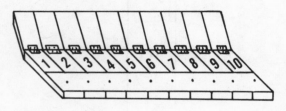

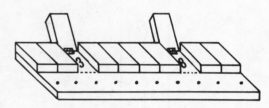

**FIG. 9-10.** Diagram of arithmetic board, with numbers covered, numbers revealed by lifting "keys," and selected opening for combined numbers or addition or subtraction. (From Latham, C. *Teaching Aids for Children with CP.* Albany, N.Y., Bureau for Physically Handicapped Children. Reproduced with permission)

**FIG. 9-11.** Traffic signs make play a useful adjunct to reality. (Courtesy R. H. Stone Products, Detroit, Mich.)

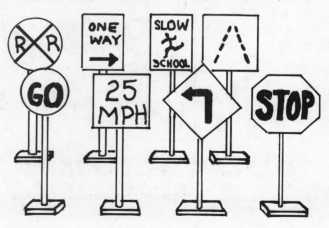

small hinges, one for each number, are "keys" the exact width of each numbered block (Fig. 9-10, *center*). When the keys are closed, the numbers are concealed. They may be raised individually to concentrate on a single number or in pairs or combinations for teaching addition or subtraction.

## OTHER AIDS

Toy catalogs contain many games involving numbers, such as Jumbo dominoes. The magnetic conversation board can also be used for this purpose.

# VISUAL AIDS FOR LEARNING

Visual aids can bring samples of real life into the classroom in pleasurable ways that are also educating.

## TRAFFIC SIGNS

Traffic signs in the home or playroom or school (Fig. 9-11) can teach the child to recognize and heed such signs on the street. Set up "traffic signs" for crawling traffic, bike traffic, wheelchair and walker traffic, or school bus orientation.

## COMMUNITY HELPERS FIGURES

A set of cut-out figures on stands (Fig. 9-12) can teach the child about family life and the various people in the community with whom he will have frequent contact. He can make them act out their roles or make up stories about them. They are a racially mixed group so that the child may learn to respect and appreciate the contributions of all people in the community.

### Sources

R. H. Stone Products
General Learning Corporation (The Judy Company) (Other Judy figures are also available for civics, story telling, and language development.)

## SEE-QUEES READING AIDS

Part puzzle and part story (Fig. 9-13), the See-Quees are made in social study topics such as Going to School, A Trip to the Zoo, The Story of Milk, Grocery Shopping, and Building a House.

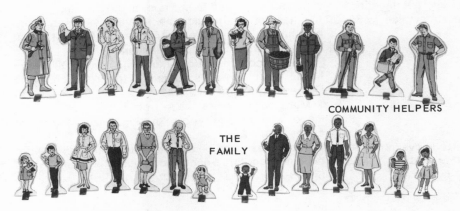

**FIG. 9-12.** Stand-up, cut-out figures of community helpers and family members. (Courtesy of R. H. Stone Products, Detroit, Mich.)

**FIG. 9-13.** See-Quees Reading Aids. Story is told by series of pictures. (Courtesy of R. H. Stone Products, Detroit,

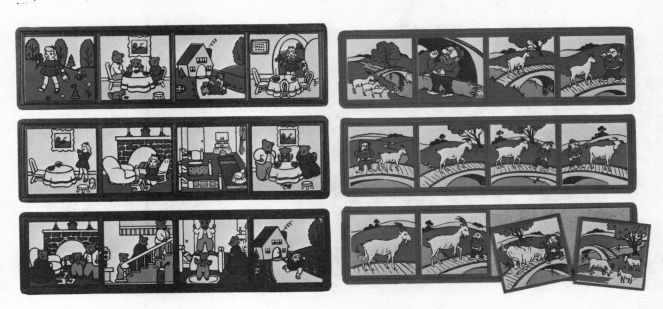

**Source**

R. H. Stone Products

## PLAYSKOOL VILLAGE FOR COMMUNITY STUDY

The child can learn about his community by building a village on the canvas street plan of the Playskool Village (Fig. 9-14). Parts of buildings are supplied to make houses, a school, city hall, church, and other buildings. And there are trees and automobiles, making a total of 120 pieces. The street plan is 32 inches square.

**Source**

Playskool—A Milton Bradley Co.

## CLOCKS

A special geared clock of large size is available for teaching the child to tell time (Fig. 9-15). "Miniclocks" are also available for individual use.

**Source**

R. H. Stone Products

## PUZZLES

Numerous puzzles are available, varying from simple to complex. A basic form is the Playskool Postal Station (Fig. 9-16) into which the "mail" in the form of beads and blocks is dropped through matching slots and recovered from a door at the bottom.

A test of imagination and perception is a more complex animal puzzle of 15 animals (Fig. 9-17) that can be put together to form a square.

Puzzles comprising common objects (Fig. 9-18) are based on color cues; others (Fig. 9-19) on basic shapes in two dimensions.

More complex are those from which patterns are made with parquetry blocks (Fig. 9-20) and color cubes (Fig. 9-21).

Puzzles can also be used to teach fractions or word building from three-dimensional kinesthetic alphabets (Fig. 9-22).

**FIG. 9-14.** Playskool Village. Child creates the buildings from various parts and lays out the town on street plan provided. (Courtesy of R. H. Stone Products, Detroit, Mich.)

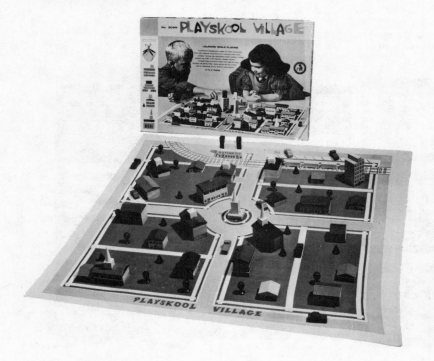

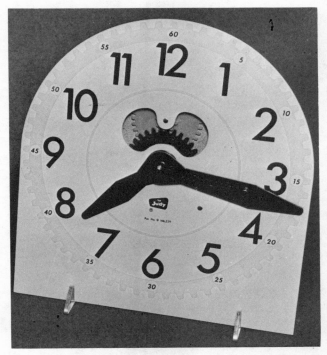

FIG. 9-15. Special clocks for learning to tell time. (Courtesy of R. H. Stone Products, Detroit, Mich.)

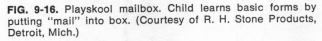

FIG. 9-16. Playskool mailbox. Child learns basic forms by putting "mail" into box. (Courtesy of R. H. Stone Products, Detroit, Mich.)

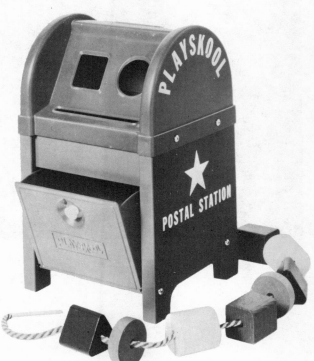

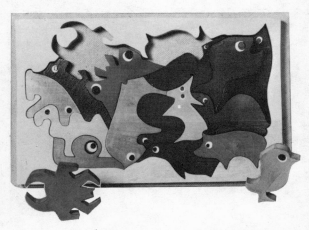

FIG. 9-17. Animal puzzle. Intricacy of puzzle teaches recognition of complex shapes. (Courtesy of R. H. Stone Products, Detroit, Mich.)

FIG. 9-18. Color-cue puzzle of common objects. (Courtesy of R. H. Stone Products, Detroit, Mich.)

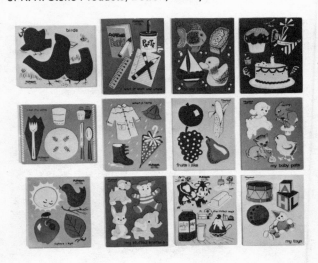

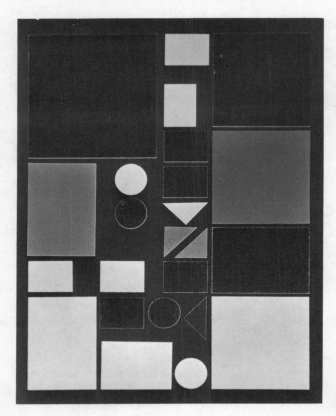

**FIG. 9-19.** Puzzle of basic shapes in two dimensions. (Courtesy of R. H. Stone Products, Detroit, Mich.)

**FIG. 9-20.** More complicated puzzle of parquetry blocks to teach form. (Courtesy of R. H. Stone Products, Detroit, Mich.)

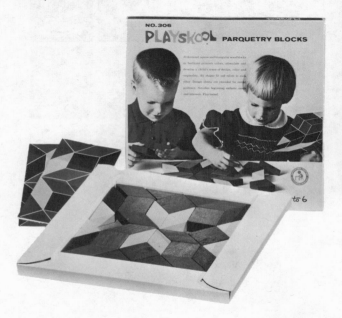

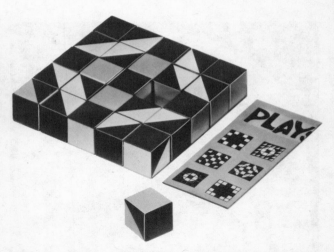

**FIG. 9-21.** Puzzle of color cubes, to teach both color recognition and form. (Courtesy of R. H. Stone Products, Detroit, Mich.)

**FIG. 9-22.** Three-dimensional kinesthetic alphabet for word-building. (Courtesy of R. H. Stone Products, Detroit, Mich.)

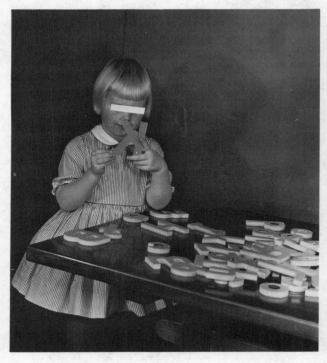

## Source

R. H. Stone Products

## AIDS FOR READING

### VISUAL SCREENING DEVICES FOR PRESCHOOL CHILDREN

Parents and those who work with children should need no reminder that good vision is essential and that the preschool child's eyes should be checked. There are aids available for group programs to screen children's eyesight so that any abnormalities may be called to the attention of the physician.

### P253 PRESCHOOL VISION SCREENING

This booklet discusses screening programs and how to go about having volunteers set them up (Fig. 9-23 and 9-24).

### Source

National Society for the Prevention of Blindness

### G116 CHARLIE BROWN DETECTIVE

This book explains to parents about early detection of children's eye problems. A single copy is free.

### Source

National Society for Prevention of Blindness

### OTHER AIDS

Several other booklets in the same program are also helpful:

G 106, *Crossed Eyes,* stresses necessity for early treatment.

G 107, *Make Sure Your Child Has Two Good Eyes,* emphasizes the importance of early eye examinations.

G 109, *The Case of the Lazy Eye,* describes various forms of amblyopia in lay terms for parents.

G 111, *This . . . Not This,* discusses the advantages of safety lenses over regular lenses.

G 113, *Who Are They?* deals with the problems of the partially seeing.

G 507, *TV and Your Eyes,* provides rules for good lighting.

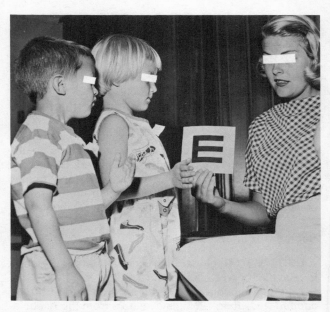

**FIG. 9-23.** Vision screening for preschool children. (Courtesy of the National Society for the Prevention of Blindness, Inc., New York)

**FIG. 9-24.** Diagram of "E" chart, used in vision screening. (Courtesy of the National Society for the Prevention of Blindness, Inc., New York)

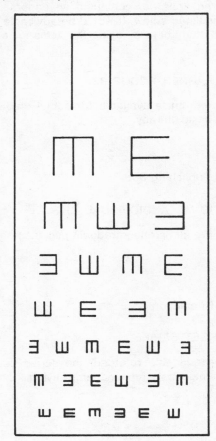

**Source**

National Society for the Prevention of Blindness

## READING AIDS FOR HANDICAPPED CHILDREN

A network of 10 regional centers was established by the U.S. Office of Education to aid teachers to improve the basic education of the disabled. Educators, supervisors, administrators, researchers, and related personnel are invited to fill out registration forms in advance of requests for materials or information.

### Sources for Information

USOE/MSU Regional Instructional Materials Center for Handicapped Children and Youth

A helpful bibliography, *Reading Aids for the Handicapped* (rev. June 1966), is available from the Association of Hospital and Institution Libraries.

## SIMPLIFIED READING MATERIAL FOR TEENAGERS AND ADULTS

Several sources are available for older persons. This listing does not constitute an endorsement for any items listed below. It would be advisable to make a careful study before buying the items for a specific person.

SLOW LEARNER PROGRAM

This program is available for social studies, English, and basic literacy.

**Source**

Follett Publishing Co.

EDUCATIONAL AUDIOVISUAL KITS

These are film strips introducing science and social studies.

**Source**

Curtis Circulation Co.

THE TARGET SERIES

For the educable retarded, the series deals with employment, citizenship, and family living.

**Source**

Mafex Associates, Inc.

SCRIPTOGRAPHIC TEACHING AIDS

These booklets and transparencies comprise illustrated units of information.

**Source**

Channing L. Bete Co., Inc.

LAUBACH LITERACY MATERIALS

These materials provide beginning reading for English-speaking adults.

**Source**

New Readers Press (Division of Laubach Literacy, Inc.)

LARGE PRINT MATERIALS

Texts, test materials, and fiction through adulthood are provided in large print.

**Source**

National Association for the Visually Handicapped

NEW YORK TIMES LARGE TYPE WEEKLY

This is a 24-page tabloid printed in jumbo type for adults.

**Source**

Large Type Weekly, New York Times

SCOPE

This publication has articles and stories edited for a 4- to 6-grade reading level, but the content is at the 8- to 12-grade interest level.

**Source**

*Scholastic Magazine* and Book Services

# 10
# Continuing Education for Young Adults

The young adult, even though handicapped, will find a number of opportunities available for continuing his education, whether this be vocational training or college work leading to a degree, with employment opportunities requiring such advanced training.

## EDUCATION BY TELEPHONE

The new educational method which brings the school to the student has been used successfully by some severely disabled readers of *Rehabilitation Gazette.* It is the School-to-Home telephone equipment developed by Executone, Inc., and furnished by the Bell Telephone System and independent companies nationally. The student at home is provided with an electronic intercommunication unit similar to the types used in offices but specially engineered for use with telephone lines. He speaks through the home unit by pressing the "talk-bar." His voice carries over private telephone lines and is received by the unit in the classroom. He hears the discussions in the classroom between his teacher and the other students. He "attends" school. Unlike correspondence courses, telephone work counts toward residence requirements. For some, trying it in high school has been the bridge leading to college.

Eager students report that the cost of using such a unit is less than that for transportation to a school or college. The costs depend upon the established rates in the area and the distance involved. Most state education departments accept this method, and more than 38 states reimburse for part or all of the cost. The Veterans Administration has also financed telephone studies for some.

The leader of the crusade for education by telephone is J. A. Richards, Educational Director of Executone, Inc. He is chairman of the Education for the Handicapped by Telephone Committee. One of the main objectives of the committee is to work with handicapped students in persuading schools and colleges to enroll severely disabled students.

### Source for Information

For personal assistance and information on techniques, costs, and financing, and suggestions for overcoming initial professional skepticism, write to:
Executone, Inc., Special Education Division
J. A. Richards, Educational Director

# CORRESPONDENCE STUDY

Correspondence study has been an exciting adventure for many *Rehabilitation Gazette* readers. Many have combined it with attendance by telephone or in person to finish high school or complete a college degree. Others have achieved specific vocational goals, such as accounting or creative writing, and are now earning substantial incomes at home. Many take one or two courses a year for the sheer delight of systematic learning.

If you have not tried correspondence study, we suggest you send for the National University Extension Association Guide and write to the universities and colleges listed for catalogs on the subjects which most intrigue you.

### Source for Information

National University Extension Association

### CREDIT

No accredited college or university in the United States will grant a degree on the basis of correspondence alone. A few state boards, colleges, and universities either do not accept correspondence credits or grant them only limited recognition. If you plan to take courses for credit in an academic program, obtain the approval of your own board or institution before registering.

### RESIDENCE REQUIREMENTS

Most institutions have set limitations on the amount of correspondence study that may be applied toward a degree; the maximum at any institution is the equivalent of two years of credit. Typically, credit earned by correspondence study may not be used toward an advanced degree. No university or college requires less than one year of residence study for a degree. However, "attendance" by telephone often does fulfill residence requirements.

### SPECIAL SERVICES

Some correspondence departments provide services, such as courses in Braille and recordings. Some individual instructors at the various colleges will accept study assignments on tape.

### FEES

Check with your state vocational rehabilitation office for advice and financial assistance. Some universities have limited funds available for tuition and scholarships.

### ACCREDITED INSTITUTIONS

Fifty-two colleges are members of the National University Extension Association and offer full programs of correspondence study. For a fascinating list of the hundreds of different courses offered by accredited American colleges and universities, consult the *Guide to Correspondence Study.*

### Source for Information

National University Extension Association

### OVERSEAS REGISTRATIONS

Many of the courses given in the United States are available to those outside continental United States at a very slightly higher rate. There may be in your country a sponsored project through which you may receive UNESCO gift coupons to use for home-study tuition at the University of Chicago and other universities.

**Source for Information**

UNESCO Gift Coupon Office

## UNACCREDITED INSTITUTIONS

There are a number of unaccredited correspondence schools, otherwise known as "diploma factories," that foist worthless degrees on the unwary. The National Home Study Council lists the accredited private home study schools and will send their list on request.

**Source for Information**

National Home Study Council

See also the article "Home Study Courses," by J. Kelly in the *Journal of Rehabilitation,* Volume 32, pages 22–23, 1966.

## COLLEGE ATTENDANCE FOR DISABLED STUDENTS

Wheelchairs on campus are no longer a novelty (Fig. 10-1). As a result of many inquiries, useful information on college resources for disabled students was compiled by *Rehabilitation Gazette:* Most colleges attended by wheelchair students have revealed a deep interest in the problems of the disabled by eliminating as many barriers as possible. Many have installed ramps or have moved classrooms to tailor their older buildings to rolling students. Most colleges are planning their newer buildings with the disabled student in mind. Following are four universities that are especially adapted to accommodate the wheelchair student and one geared to the home-bound or hospitalized student.

## UNIVERSITY OF ILLINOIS

A number of years ago, Timothy J. Nugent started a "temporary" rehabilitation program for eight disabled men students. In 1961 there were 163 disabled students; 101 were in wheelchairs. Thanks to his great personal drive, he has inspired the government and several organizations to donate funds so that almost every building on campus is ramped and accessible. The disabled students have access to every curriculum on campus and are able to participate fully in all campus activities. They even have their own fraternity, Delta Sigma Omicron.

There is a fleet of four buses equipped with hydraulic lifts which make hourly trips around campus,

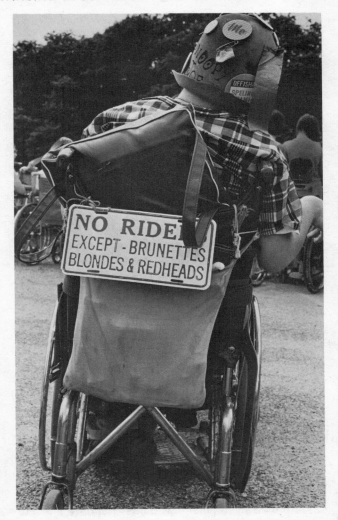

**FIG. 10-1.** A sense of humor is communication at its best. (Courtesy of United Cerebral Palsy of Nassau County, Roosevelt, New York)

dropping students off at their academic classes and physical therapy classes, which are attended by every rehabilitation student in place of physical education. The buses also take the students shopping.

The University is the focus of many college representatives. The U.S. Office of Vocational Rehabilitation is financing their visits to campus to encourage their participation in similar programs.

## SOUTHERN ILLINOIS UNIVERSITY

Since 1958 this University has been similarly modifying its physical facilities and administrative and academic procedures to enable severely disabled persons to enroll in college and graduate school and to take part in campus functions. In 1960 there were 63 such students; 32 were in wheelchairs.

Special mention should be made of the Vocational Technical Institute of the University, providing two-year programs leading to associate degrees in such fields as accounting, drafting, and retail sales, in which many disabled students are enrolled.

## UNIVERSITY OF MISSOURI

In the fall of 1962 the University enrolled disabled students. The U.S. Office of Vocational Rehabilitation selected it for a five-year research and demonstration project in the education of disabled college students. It will serve Region 6, comprising the seven-state area of Missouri, Iowa, Minnesota, North and South Dakota, Nebraska, and Kansas. Elevators and ramps have been installed.

## UNIVERSITY OF CALIFORNIA AT LOS ANGELES

The UCLA program for disabled students was established soon after World War II, when many veterans resumed their education. Practically every building has adjacent parking, ramps, elevators, and special restrooms and telephones. The Office of Special Services offers special vocational and educational services. The Will Rogers Memorial Scholarship is available only to disabled students.

## RELIGIOUS EDUCATION

For the disabled person who does not have a pastor to assist him, advice on religious education and pastoral counseling is available.

### Source for Information

Postgraduate Center for Mental Health
Dept. of Community Services and Education

## REFERENCES

### College Education for the Handicapped

*College Level Examination Program.* Educational Testing Service, Box 592, Princeton, N.J. 08540. (Information and list of testing centers where tests translate self-acquired knowledge into college credits)

Hall, R. E., Lehman, E. F. *Directory: Some Colleges and Universities with Special Facilities to Accommodate Handicapped Students.* Washington, D.C., Office of Education, Department of Health, Education, and Welfare, 1966. (Contains over 150 colleges listed relative to on-campus ramps, classroom ramps, library ramps, beveled curbs, reserved parking, modified toilets.)

"Higher education and employment," *Rehabilitation Gazette,* Vol. 10, 1967.

Kelly, J. "Home study courses," J Rehab 32:22, 1966.

Rusalem, H. "Guiding the physically handicapped college student," Rehab Lit 23:275, 1962. (Resources for counseling that will make the experience more realistic)

Tucker, W. "Rehabilitation and higher education," Rehab Counsel Bull 6:18, 1963. (Campus problems and relation of education to employment potential)

### School and Career Guides

Adams, W., Garraty, J.A. *A Guide to Study Abroad.* Des Moines, Meredith Press, 1967. (Comprehensive handbook for teachers, students, and guidance counselors who plan to study in Europe, Latin America, or the Near or Far East).

*American Universities and Colleges,* 9th ed., 1964; *American Junior Colleges,* 6th ed., 1963; *Fellowships in the Arts and Sciences,* 10th ed., 1967–68; *A Guide to Graduate Study: Programs Leading to the Ph.D. Degree,* 3rd ed., 1965. Washington, D.C., American Council on Education.

Angel, J. *How & Where to Get Scholarships and Loans,* New York, Regents Pub. Co., Inc., 1964.

Hall, L. D. *Financial Aid for the Graduate Student,* College Opportunity Inc. 1971–1972.

Herman, Shirley Yvonne. *Guide to Study in Europe,* Four Winds Press, 1969.

Keeslar O. *A National Catalog of Scholarships for Students Entering College.* Dubuque, Iowa, William C. Brown, Co., 3rd Ed. 1967.

Lovejoy, C. E. *Lovejoy's College Guide,* 11th ed. New York, Simon & Schuster, 1970.

Maxwell, B. G., *Financial Aids for Undergraduate Students,* College Opportunity Inc., 1968.

McKee, R. *Financial Assistance for College Students.* Washington, D.C. Superintendent of Documents, U.S. Government Printing Office, 1965. Lists amounts, number of scholarships, loans, employment opportunities, and other financial assistance at more than 2,000 colleges and universities. (Present supply exhausted—check local library)

*Need a Lift?* American Legion, Americanism Division, Indianapolis, Ind. (Annually revised handbook published as part of the American Legion's Education and Scholarship Program to assist students, parents, and counselors to secure current information on careers and scholarships. 25 cents.)

Renetzky A., *Annual Registry of Grant Support 1971.* Orange, N.J., Academic Media, 1971.

Sabo, A., ed. *College Facts and Financial Aid.* Monrovia, N.Y., Chronicle Guidance Publications, 1970 (A comprehensive series, 5 volumes plus supplementary bulletins, revised annually and designed to provide a library of basic information on scholarships, college selection, costs and major areas of study)

*Study Abroad,* Vol. 19, New York, UNESCO Publications Center, 1972–1974 (Contains latest information on over 250,000 scholarships and fellowships in 116 countries; also opportunities for foreign students to study in the United States)

Turner, D. R. *College Scholarships*. New York, Arco Publishing Company.

*Vacation Study Abroad*, Vol. 19. New York, UNESCO Publications Center, 1971 (Contains a list of 1,000 educational and cultural vacation suggestions, such as summer university courses, study tours, work campus, and other opportunities which include sightseeing and study activities; also scholarship and financial assistance for summer programs of this type)

### Educational Opportunities for Handicapped

Arthur, J. K. "Pros and Cons of College," In *Employment for the Handicapped: A Guide for Disabled, Their Families and Their Counselors,* Nashville, Tenn. Abrington Press, 1967.

*For the Disabled—Help Through Vocational Rehabilitation.* Washington, D.C., Social and Rehabilitation Services, Department of Health, Education, and Welfare. (Available free)

*A Guide to Federally Supported Programs.* Washington, D.C., Division of Student Financial Aid, Bureau of Higher Education, U.S. Office of Education. (Free reference folder containing detailed information on scholarships, grants, loans, and other aid)

Tucker, W. V., Waters, H. J., "Higher Education and Handicapped Students," 1964. (Handbook available free from Dr. Waters, Kansas State Teachers College, Emporia, Kans. 66801. Tabulates facilities for the handicapped in U.S. colleges)

"Wheelchairs on Campus—Performance," Washington, D.C., President's Committee on Employment of the Handicapped, 1966.

### Religious Education

*Bibliographies for Parents and Teachers of Retarded Children.* National Association for Retarded Children, Arlington, Tex. 76011 (Protestant, Jewish and Catholic)

"Rehabilitation Literature," National Easter Seal Society for Crippled Children and Adults. (See index for abstracts of articles on religion in the journal)

### Sex Education and Family Life

Calderwood, Deryk. *About Your Sexuality*. Boston, Beacon Press, 1972. (A curriculum for sex educators to present to teenagers.)

Gordon, S. *Facts About Sex for Exceptional Youth*. Plainview, N.Y. Charles Brown, Inc., 1969.

Gordon S. *Facts About Sex: A Basic Guide*. New York, John Day Co., 1970.

Hinton, G. D. *Teaching Sex Education: A Guide for Teachers*. Palto Alto, Calif., Fearon Brothers, 1969.

Hudson, M. W. *All About Me: Girl's Book*. Lawrence, Kans., University of Kansas, Special Education Instructional Materials Center, 1966.

Hudson, M. W. *All About Me: Girl's Book*. Lawrence, Kans., Univ. of Kansas, Special Educational Instructional Materials Center, 1966.

Johnson, Eric, *Love and Sex in Plain Language*. New York, rev. 2nd ed, J. B. Lippincott, Co., 1967.

Julian, C. J., and Jackson, E. N. *Modern Sex Education for Highschoolers*. New York, Holt, Rinehart, 1967.

*Resource Guide in Sex Education for Mentally Retarded*. A Joint Project of SIECUS and American Association for Health, Physical Education, and Recreation, Washington, D.C. and SIECUS, New York, 1971. (Includes reading and audiovisual resources.)

Trenkle, C. *You*. Lawrence, Kans., University of Kansas, Special Education Instructional Materials Center, 1966.

Schults, Gladys (Denny) *Letters to a new generation; for Todays inquiring teenage girl,* New York, J. B. Lippincott, Co., 1971.

# IV
# RECREATION

# 11
# Children's Recreation Aids

Recreation emphasizes the constructive use of leisure time (Fig. 11-1). At all ages, leisure time may be spent in group situations, in partnership exchanges, or at solitary interests. The importance of a planned play environment cannot be overemphasized, and this is especially so in the care of the disabled child. From infancy on, situations must be contrived to promote learning and physical development—handling, sorting, pushing, pulling, climbing, walking, and body control.

While recreation aids for the handicapped are few at present, they will increase over the years as suggestions come from readers. This chapter discusses only items found specifically useful to persons with cerebral palsy. It is recognized, however, that many of these individuals can make use of the many existing resources for those with other disabilities.

## Sources for Information

American Association for Health, Physical Education and Recreation

Bureau of Outdoor Recreation

National Recreation and Park Association

National Easter Seal Society for Crippled Children and Adults

Southern Regional Education Board

United Cerebral Palsy Associations, Inc.

See references at the end of this chapter for a full list of publications available from these and other sources.

## TOYS AND GAMES

Toys cannot be classified or selected by age groups. Rather, they should be chosen for the developmental purpose that they may serve for the disabled child; the highest enjoyment is that which is meaningful.

### Precautions

1. Choose sturdy toys that do not break when dropped or that do not come apart when handled clumsily.
2. Be sure lead-free, nonpoisonous paints were used.
3. Check to see that the toy is smoothly finished and that no metal or plastic edges or corners are sharp enough to cut or pierce.

4. Be sure the toy can be sterilized and washed easily and effectively.
5. Select toys easy to handle and easy to grasp.
6. Make certain that the parts of a toy fit carefully. For example, a peg should go easily into a hole but should not fall out because the hole is too shallow or too wide in diameter.
7. Avoid the use of buttons for eyes on animal toys or dolls.
8. Remember that dark versus light or contrasting colors provide the best visibility. For example, the "well" of a puzzle into which parts are placed should be darker or lighter than the topboard that holds the pieces (Fig. 11-2).
9. On home-made toys, add a hard finish enamel with an overcoating of spar varnish to furnish a durable surface for toys that need frequent washing.

### Sources for Information

The United Cerebral Palsy Association Bulletin, *Recreation for the Homebound,* suggests the following sources for toys. See also, the references section, under Toys and Games.

Association for Childhood Education International

**FIG. 11-1.** Learning to "dance" as a form of exercise. This is one example of constructive use of leisure time. (Courtesy of United Cerebral Palsy of Nassau County, New York)

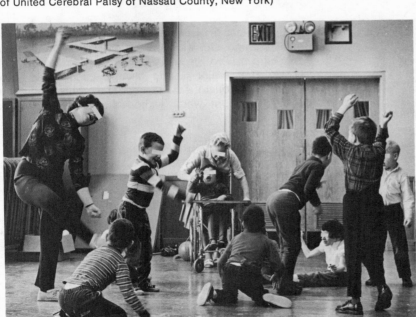

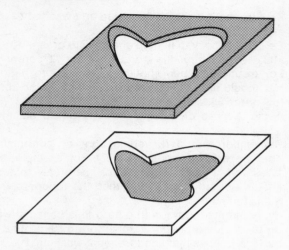

**FIG. 11-2.** Contrasting parts of a puzzle for easy visibility.

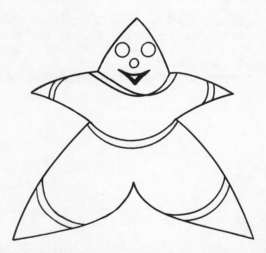

**FIG. 11-3.** Star-shaped bean bag, for easy grasping.

**FIG. 11-4** Giant foam blocks, easily handled, with a variety of shapes and colors. (Courtesy of Creative Playthings, Inc., Princeton, N.J., and Los Angeles, Calif.)

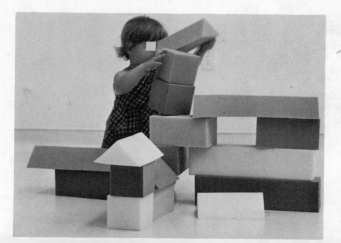

Warren Paper-Built-rite Toys
Community Playthings
Constructive Playthings
Creative Playthings
Kenner Products
R. H. Stone Products (Mor-Play Catalog)

### STAR BEAN BAG

Tossing a bean bag provides good fun for young children. One that can be easily made is the star bean bag (Fig. 11-3). Its points make it easy for children to grasp.

**Construction**

1. Cut out star shape from any sturdy material. Any size bag is acceptable; suggested proportions are 9 inches from head to toe, with a 3-inch-wide waist-line.
2. Sew up except for a small opening to turn to right side and to stuff.
3. Trim in any way you please. A doll's face can be made on a widely cut point, with other points as hands and feet.
4. Stuff with a quantity of dried beans that will leave a loose, flexible feeling to the bag, and sew up the hole.

### CRYSTAL ORCHESTRA

Eight water glasses can be turned into music makers. Fill them with water to the proper levels to make one octave. Tap the glasses with a pencil to get the notes. Then paint a ring around each glass (with bright nail polish) so they can be refilled with the right amount of water without having to be tested every time.

### BABY-SEE MIRROR

Psychologists say that infancy is the crucial time of learning; the toys the infant plays with can promote that learning. A child's interest and wonder at his own reflection can be easily seen and stimulated with a baby safe mirror.

**Source**

Creative Playthings, Inc.

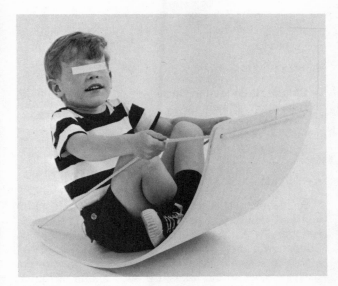

FIG. 11-5. Rocky Board. Exercise and fun. (Courtesy of Creative Playthings, Inc., Princeton, N.J., and Los Angeles, Calif.)

## GIANT FOAM BLOCKS

Easy-to-grasp blocks (Fig. 11-4) of foam help the toddler learn to handle objects, and sort and fit as he plays.

**Source**

Creative Playthings, Inc.

## ROCKY BOARD

Curved board with rope handles on the sides (Fig. 11-5) can take a child on many a imaginary trip. At the same time he is learning to push and pull.

**Source**

Creative Playthings, Inc.

## CIRCULAR RUBBER PUZZLES

The simplicity of outline of the objects in these puzzles (Fig. 11-6) help the child to see their relationships and to make distinctions between them by fitting them into the proper circles.

**Source**

Creative Playthings, Inc.

## TUNNEL OF FUN

Promoting physical activity and body control, the crawl-through Tunnel of Fun (Fig. 11-7) helps kindergarten age children gain a sense of personal mastery.

**Source**

Creative Playthings, Inc.

# BACKYARD AND PLAYGROUND EQUIPMENT

Outdoor recreation is as essential to the handicapped child as to others, and many types of equipment can be adapted to his needs. The first playground specifically designed for disabled children was completed in 1960 for the United Cerebral Palsy Center of Nassau County, New York (Fig. 11-8). It was developed by the Playground Corporation of America. Since then, the Playground Corporation has carried on considerable research and has incorporated its findings in the "playscapes" it has designed for other handicapped children's facilities.

Not all equipment has to be made especially for handicapped children. Selection may be made by considering the developmental needs and interests of the group and consulting reliable toy companies for durable and safe equipment.

FIG. 11-6. Circular rubber puzzles, for experience in distinguishing shapes. (Courtesy of Creative Playthings, Inc., Princeton, N.J., and Los Angeles, Calif.)

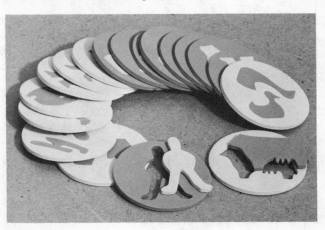

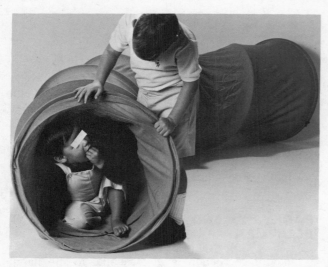

**FIG. 11-7.** Tunnel of Fun. A game of I-spy is just one of many to which this toy lends itself. (Courtesy of Creative Playthings, Inc., Princeton, N.J., and Los Angeles, Calif.)

**FIG. 11-8.** "Playscape" especially designed for disabled children, featuring equipment that is both fun and outdoor exercise. (Courtesy of United Cerebral Palsy of Nassau County, New York)

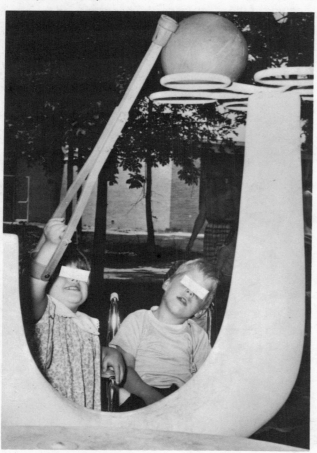

**Sources for Information**

Childcraft Education Corp.
Community Playthings
Constructive Playthings
Playground Corp.
Bureau of Outdoor Recreation

## MODIFIED OBSTACLE COURSE

Backyard play equipment (Figs. 11-9 and 11-10) adapted from an obstacle course designed by Carol Hatcher, Ph.D., Chairman of the Department of Special Education at Los Angeles State College, has proved highly successful for use by children with cerebral palsy. Almost all the items are adaptations of regular playground equipment for nursery age children. In addition to the equipment, the ground surface has been specially prepared with gravel and irregular turf to provide experiences in walking on varied surface.

## THE SKYRIDE

A device currently being used in the preschool nursery of the United Cerebral Palsy Center for children 18 months to 4 years of age, in Van Nuys, California, is an overhead cable with a handhold with pulleys called a Skyride (Fig. 11-11). It was designed by Rudy Diamond, speech therapist and teacher of the deaf. The Skyride is not only delightful recreation for the children but is therapeutically useful in providing:

1. A motivating bilateral activity for the lower extremities, in which both ambulatory and nonambulatory patients enjoy walking back and forth when their feet are touching the ground while the upper extremities are supported by the pulleys
2. Bilateral hand use for hemiplegics, with reach and grasp required
3. An extremely motivating activity
4. Perceptual stimulation, with awareness of the body in space
5. Bilateral stretch in shoulders and arms

### Construction

The skyride is fairly simple to make and can be set up in an outside play area or a large therapy room. The equipment may be attached to a tree, fence, or any solid backing.

The diagram (Fig. 11-12) shows the dimensions and materials used.

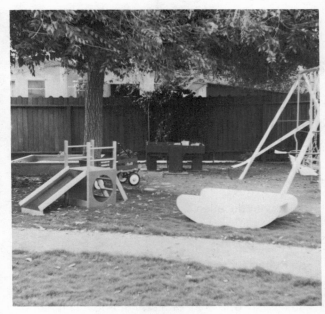

**FIG. 11-9.** Modified obstacle course has small steps with slide and crawl hole; two sandboxes, one on the ground and one standing; a set of swings; and a rocking "boat." (Courtesy of P. Holser-Buehler, UCPA United Cerebral Palsy)

**FIG. 11-10.** Modified obstacle course consisting of crawl-through barrel, practice steps of different heights, stepping stones painted different colors, parallel bars, and a large platform with steps, a ramp, and a slide. (Courtesy of P. Holser-Buehler, UCPA of Los Angeles)

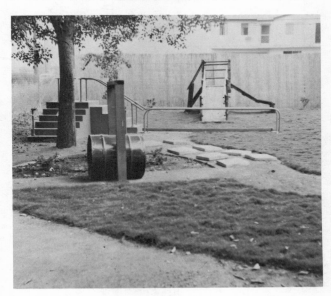

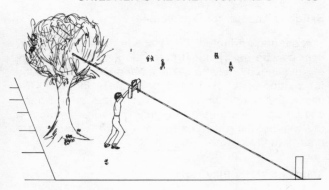

**FIG. 11-11.** Skyride. Thrilling form of recreation provides excellent exercise and stimulation. (Courtesy of F. Yossem, United Cerebral Palsy Prenursery, Van Nuys, Calif.)

**FIG. 11-12.** Diagram for construction of Skyride. Dimensions are in inches. *Top, left,* cross-section, side view, of riding section, showing dimensions and location of cable and pulleys. *Top, right,* cross section, end view of riding section, showing locations of bolts. *Bottom,* completed Skyride, showing dimensions; detail *A* shows doweling of grab bar. Drawing is to scale 1" = 4". (Courtesy of F. Yossem, United Cerebral Palsy Prenursery, Van Nuys, Calif.)

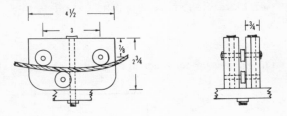

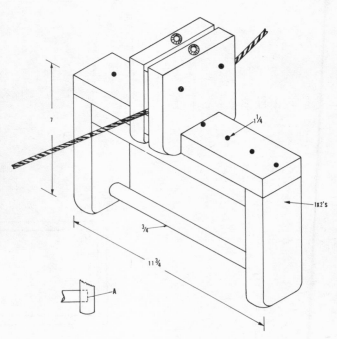

### Sandbox Adapter for Wheelchair

A sandbox adapted to the needs of the wheelchair user can be easily constructed (Fig. 11-13). The legs of the sandbox may be partly embedded in the ground for outdoor use or placed on casters indoors. The physically handicapped child confined to a wheelchair must have ample play space when reaching in the sandbox, and for this reason *length* is much more important than width.

### Sand and Water Play Table

A suitable table for play in sand and water is commercially available. Dimensions should be specified when ordering.

### Source

Community Playthings

### ROCKING TUB

A tub with a rounded bottom becomes a round-bottom boat for youngsters sailing an imaginary ocean (Fig. 11-14). More than shared fun, the toy offers balance practice.

### Precautions

1. Have child wear headguard to protect him against tipping.
2. With youngsters who are very unstable, pad the rim of the tub with foam held on by wide tape, to protect against bruising or knocking the teeth against the rim.
3. Better still, get the toy in plastic composition to avoid the hazards of bruising (example: Rock-n-Spin of Childcraft)

### Source

Childcraft Education Corp.

### SUPER-TUBE

The Super-Tube is really an inner tube used for airplanes. It is a seating joy—six small children can sit in it for a singing spree. It can also be used for a punching bag, or a float, or a swing. And it is great for tumbling, when placed on a mat.

A combination of auto, truck, and airplane tubes can create a large play structure with limitless variations. Arranged in different ways they become forts, castles, houses, or tunnels.

**FIG. 11-13.** Diagram for construction of sandbox adapted for wheelchair user. *Top,* side view, showing ground level; *bottom,* top view.

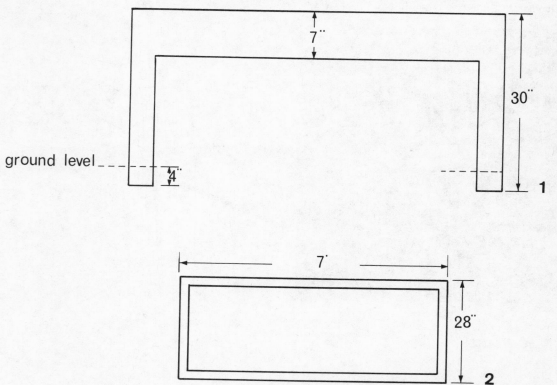

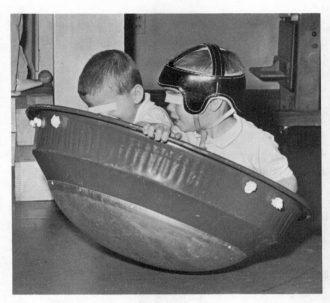

FIG. 11-14. Tub-like roller-rocker. The two "men" in the tub gain practice in balance while "sailing" a linoleum "sea." (Courtesy of Cerebral Palsy Center of Montgomery County, Md.)

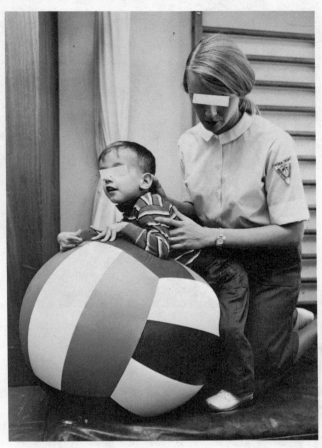

## Source

Tubes are available from most surplus stores, local air fields, or rubber manufacturers. The "Bouncing Tube" is commercially available from:
J. A. Preston Corp.

## URETHANE FOAM FORMS FOR TUMBLING

Firm urethane foam in a variety of shapes, encased in Hypalon-coated nylon fabrics, can be used both for movement and for play.

## Source

Skill Development Equipment, Co.

## INFLATABLE PLASTIC BALL

Large, inflatable plastic balls make excellent toys and are useful for therapy (Fig. 11-15).

## Sources

Ideal Toy Corp.
Spielwaren-Hemmeler AG

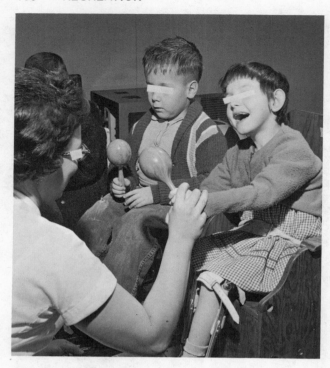

**FIG. 11-16.** Specially built chairs to provide security and relaxation for children at play. (Courtesy of Children's Hospital School, Eugene, Ore.)

**FIG. 11-17.** Cut-out table with stand-in boxes, giving support and freedom for arms in group play. (A. Slominski, ORT, Indiana University Medical Center)

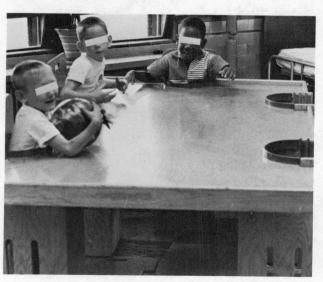

## INFLATABLE RUBBER BALL

Rubber balls which inflate from 44 inches to 67 inches in circumference are also available.

**Source**

Sun Products Corp.

# EQUIPMENT FOR SMALL GROUP ACTIVITIES

Although the child needs to learn to play alone, group activity is also essential for full development. Many of the items already suggested are suitable for group activity. Others are given here.

### SPECIAL CHAIRS

Chairs should be designed to fit the children and should be supplied with footstools or supports at functional levels (Fig. 11-16). Seat belts at the lower hip level, like auto safety belts, provide security and allow for the relaxation needed during play. See also the section on Sitting and Standing Equipment in Chapter 1.

### STAND-IN TABLE

A stand-in table is excellent for group games at elbow level. The table gives support and freedom for the use of the arms (Fig. 11-17). Slots in the stand-in boxes allow air to circulate. The boxes are on rollers and can be attached to various cut-out sections of the table, allowing new play partners. See also the section on Stand-in Tables in Chapter 1.

### ROLLING BLOCK FOR GROUP GAMES

A six-sided block can easily be made (Fig. 11-18) and will provide a good group game. With numbers or different colors on the flat surfaces, the children can roll the block and guess which number or color will be on top when the block stops. The player who guesses correctly wins. A blanket on top of the table makes an ideal rolling surface. This is a good example of an adapted toy that moves but cannot go far and that has some learning value built into the fun. For other good ideas, see the booklet from which this came: *Recreation for the Mentally Retarded: A Handbook for Ward Personnel.*

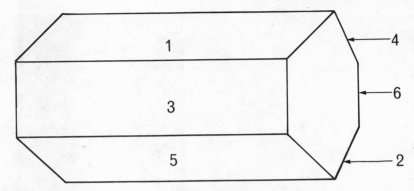

**FIG. 11-18.** Diagram of six-sided rolling block. Numbers or colors make block into a guessing game. (From Bensberg, G. J., ed. *Recreation for the Mentally Retarded: A Handbook for Ward Personnel.* Atlanta, Southern Regional Education Board, 1966. Reproduced with permission)

### Construction

1. Use 4-inch by 4-inch or 6-inch by 6-inch lumber, 12 to 18 inches long.
2. Saw to make either six or eight sides. Sides should be equal in size.
3. File the edges and corners slightly to make the block roll more freely.
4. Print a different number on each flat surface, or paint each surface with a different color.

## ADAPTED PHYSICAL EDUCATION ACTIVITIES

The handicapped child needs directed physical education if he is to be able to develop to the best of his capacity. Such training can help him to acquire good eye-and-hand coordination (Fig. 11-19), to develop arm, shoulder, and body control (Fig. 11-20), hand and arm strength and control (Fig. 11-21), and bilateral arm usage (Fig. 11-22).

The comments of those who have worked in physical education with handicapped children merit repeating here:

"Try to relate motion to the development and learning of the severely involved child."—Don Burton, United Cerebral Palsy of Denver, Colo.

"Movement is a nonverbal expression of feeling." —Barbara Mettler, Director, Tucson Creative Dance Studio, Tucson, Ariz.

"If physical education will put less emphasis on competition and use its good background of physiology of body mechanics and development, it has much to offer in varieties of noncompetitive physical activities for the physically handicapped, as well as for the retarded."—John Barringer, Director of Health, Physical Education, and Recreation of Tucson District 1 Public Schools, Tucson, Ariz.

### Sources for Information

For courses and seminars related to adapted physical education, physical fitness, corrective and adapted activities, or creative movement, contact the persons listed below. The list is by no means a complete one on the many innovative programs in the United States. Consult the uninversity or college nearest your facilities.

Bob L. Beasley, University of Southern Florida
Dr. Elmo Roundy, Brigham Young University
Delores A. Black, Bowling Green State University
Arthur G. Miller, Boston University
Walter L. Olsen, University of Arizona
E. P. Wooten, Oregon State University

### STUFFED, WEIGHTED TOY ANIMALS

For weight training and basic movement experiences, stuffed toy animals weighted with buckshot serve a good purpose and appeal to the youngsters (Fig. 11-23). Black kittens hold 7 pounds of buckshot; tigers, 10 pounds; and dogs, 15 pounds.

## EQUIPMENT FOR MUSIC-MAKING

All children enjoy music and rhythm, and can participate in making their own music at an early age (Fig. 11-24). For a rhythm band, many of the instru-

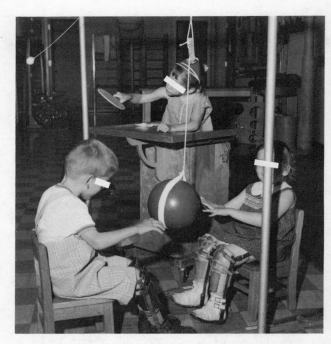

FIG. 11-19. Physical education for handicapped children: basketball suspended on a rope for catching and striking. (Courtesy of O. H. Marx, Physical Education Dept., University Hospital School, University of Iowa)

FIG. 11-20. Physical education for handicapped children: push-ups on an exercise mat. (Courtesy of O. H. Marx, Physical Education Dept., University Hospital School, University of Iowa)

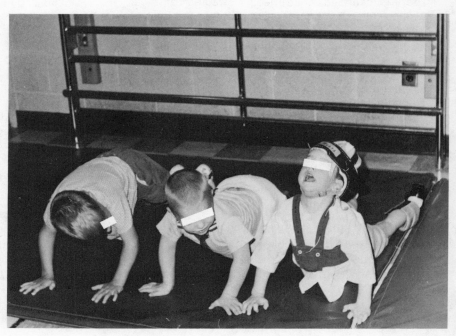

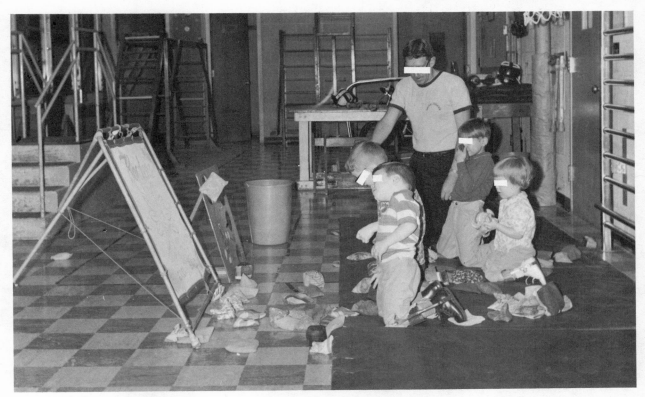

**FIG. 11-21.** Physical education for handicapped children: bean bag throwing. (Courtesy of O. H. Marx, Physical Education Dept., University Hospital School, University of Iowa)

**FIG. 11-22.** Physical education for handicapped children: an adaptation of basketball. (Courtesy of O. H. Marx, Physical Education Dept., University Hospital School, University of Iowa)

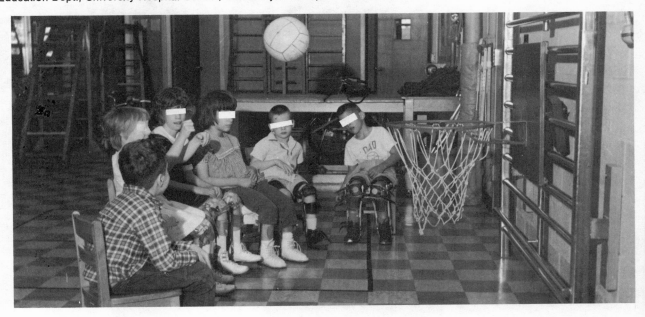

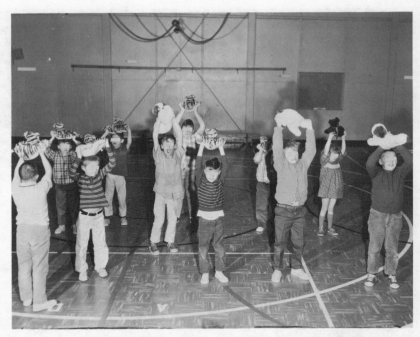

**FIG. 11-23.** Physical education for handicapped children. Weighed toy animals provide means of stretching and lifting exercise. (From Lounsberry, J. Weight training for mentally retarded at primary level. *Challenge 2:*2, 1967. Reproduced with permission)

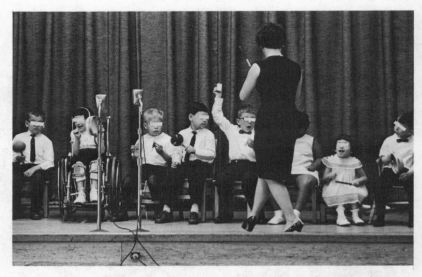

**FIG. 11-24.** Rhythm band of handicapped children. Here it's the beat that counts, but the coordination that is learned counts even more. (Courtesy of United Cerebral Palsy of Nassau County, N.Y.)

ments can be made. The following directions are from the Alpha Chi Omega Fraternity book, *Toy Book of Self-Help Toys to Make for the Handicapped*.

## MARACAS

### Construction

1. Use a small can from Kodak 35-mm film (used in Leica and similar 35-mm cameras). Drill a hole in the lid of the can, to take a screw.
2. Into the end of a piece of ¼-inch doweling, which will make the handle, drill a screw hole, using a fine drill to prevent splitting.
3. Screw a small round-head screw from the inside of the lid into the handle.
4. Sand and shellac the handle.
5. Fill the can with about 12 BB shot and screw the lid on.

## JINGLE BELLS

### Construction

1. Remove all bristles from the wire frame of a vegetable brush and paint the handle.
2. Attach six Christmas trimming bells to the wire frame with picture frame wire.

## RHYTHM STICKS

### Construction

1. Cut a broom handle into 10- or 11-inch lengths. Smooth the ends with a file or sandpaper.
2. Paint each pair of sticks a different bright color.

## DRUMS

### Construction

1. Remove the top of a No. 10 can (the type in which canned foods are supplied to restaurants and schools). Be sure to use a smooth can opener. Leave the bottom on the can.
2. Paint the can a bright color.
3. Stretch thin inner tubing or discarded drum hides from school band instruments over the opening of the can and tie tightly with strong cord.
4. For drumsticks use 2 pieces of ¼-inch doweling 8 to 10 inches long.
5. Scoop out the hole in a rubber ball washer (called

Fuller balls) to fit the end of the doweling. An alternative drumstick can be made from a Tinker Toy stick and a knob from a drumstick.

## TRIANGLE

### Construction

1. Take a piece of thin, solid metal tubing, such as an old curtain rod, to a welding shop and have a 6- to 8-inch piece of the rod filed off for a stick. Have the remainder bent into an equilateral triangle with sides approximately 6 inches.
2. Attach ribbon or braided yarn to the triangle for a handle.

## CYMBALS

### Construction

1. Punch holes into old pan lids to hold straps (one for each lid).
2. Thread leather strap through from the top and secure it on the under side.

## JINGLE CLOGS

### Construction

1. Cut ¾-inch plywood or solid wood with a power saw into a banjo or shovel shape, 3 inches by 8 inches (Fig. 11-25).
2. Sand and shellac the paddle.
3. Attach four metal washers to the paddle with a galvanized roofing nail with a large head. The metal washers should be of two sizes. The hole of the smaller size should be smaller than the head of the nail and at least one of these should be placed next to the nailhead to hold the others in place. Leave the nail head protruding enough so that the washers will be loose.

**FIG. 11-25.** Diagram of jingle clog made with metal washers around a large roofing nail in wooden paddle.

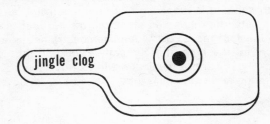
jingle clog

## TAMBOURINE

### Construction

1. Drill four holes into the top of a round metal lid from a cookie or candy box. Holes should be 1 inch from the edge of the lid.
2. Drill out the centers of eight roofing caps (shingle tins) so they will slide loosely on copper rivets.
3. Fasten the tins to the lid with four copper rivets and their washers. Place two tins and a washer on the rivet, insert into the hole, and pound the rivet with a hammer so it spreads out and is secure over the hole.

## SAND BLOCKS

### Construction

1. Make two blocks to be rubbed together. Each is approximately 1 inch by 3 or 5 inches. Sand and paint or varnish the blocks.
2. Attach a piece of coarse sand paper, 5 by 5 inches, to each block with a hand stapler.
3. Staple or nail a leather or rubber strip to each block for hand straps. Be sure the straps are loose enough for little hands.

## AID FOR TEACHING THROUGH MUSIC

An excellent program of teaching the mentally retarded through music has been established in South Carolina by the Governor's Interagency Council on Mental Retardation. The Council will make the necessary arrangements with schools or groups wishing the programs presented over closed-circuit television.

The program consists of four 30-minute video tapes, 16-mm black and white. They may be presented as singles, particularly No. 4, but for best results, they should be shown in sequence. In each of the four tapes, Dr. Richard Weber uses a different group of trainable children selected from Whitten Village, Pineland Training School, Happy Time Center, and two former pupils from New York City. With the exception of the two children on the last tape, each group is new to him and is receiving instruction, carried out in a completely unrehearsed situation, for the first time.

On the four tapes, Dr. Weber demonstrates his approach to teaching the mentally retarded through music. By utilizing a musical scale with a simple six-note range and combining letters, numbers, and other symbols, Dr. Weber shows how music becomes a motivator for developing writing and reading skills, such as left-to-right eye movement and correct visual perception, as well as self-control. The point of self-control is of great importance in the development of a self-concept by the mentally retarded child, allowing him to become aware of his surrounding environment, thus giving motivation to developing communicative skills.

Dr. Weber points out that the method requires a minimum of teacher supervision and that most special education teachers can achieve the same results that he accomplishes.

*Children Limited,* the official publication of the National Association for Retarded Children, has labeled Dr. Weber's work as setting off a revolution in the concept of teaching severely retarded children.

### Sources for Information

South Carolina Department of Mental Retardation

## REFERENCES

**Guides for Recreational Activities**

*Books on Hobbies.* Recreation Book Center, National Recreation and Park Association, Arlington, Va.

*Challenge.* American Association for Health, Physical Education and Recreation, Washington, D.C. (Newsletter published five times per year by Project on Recreation and Fitness for the Mentally Retarded)

"Day Camping for the Cerebral Palsied," Bulletin 11. United Cerebral Palsy Associations, Inc., New York. (Program guide on planning committee, resources, admission policies, program staff, equipment, transportation, costs, records)

"Frustration Versus Spontaneity: Planned Playgrounds for Handicapped Children," Playground Corporation of America, Long Island City, N.Y.

"The Future Is Yours," National Recreation and Park Association. (Brochure on careers in recreation leadership)

"Guide to Books on Recreation," Recreation Book Center, National Recreation and Park Association.

Helsel, E., Messner, S., Reid, L. *Opening New Doors to the Cerebral Palsied Through Day Care and Development Centers.* New York United Cerebral Palsy Associations, Inc. (Guide for affiliates to develop programs for the severely disabled outside the home: physical facilities, fees, programs for the children and adults, staffing, bibliography)

O'Brien, S. B. *More Than Fun.* New York, United Cerebral Palsy Associations, Inc. (Handbook of recreational programming for children and adults; community responsibility, program content, adaptations, leadership; bibliography)

"Outdoor Recreation Planning for the Handicapped," Washington, D.C., U.S. Department of the Interior, Bureau of Outdoor Recreation. (Bulletin suggesting modifications that can be made to enable handicapped children and youth to enjoy playground equipment and outdoor activities. Order from Superintendent of Documents, U.S. Government Printing Office, supply presently exhausted, check your local library.)

*Parent, Teacher and Young Child.* Arlington, Va., Recreation Book Center, National Recreation and Park Association.

*Recreation for the Handicapped in the Community Setting: A Guide.* Arlington, Va., National Recreation and Park Association. (For community recreation departments and other agencies concerned with the social and recreational needs of the handicapped, whether physically handicapped, mentally ill, or retarded)

*Recreation for the Mentally Retarded: A Handbook for Ward Personnel.* Atlanta, Ga., Southern Regional Education Board. (Developed as part of an attendant-training project. Contains active games, quiet games, music and rhythm, arts and crafts)

"Recreation for the Physically Handicapped," Chicago, Ill., National Easter Seal Society for Crippled Children and Adults, 1964. (Reference list compiled in 1963 on activities, camping, day camping, adapted physical education and crafts)

"Rehabilitation Gazette," St. Louis, Mo. (Journal written by and for the disabled, to exchange ideas for meaningful use of time)

"Swimming for the Cerebral Palsied," Bulletin 10. United Cerebral Palsy Associations, Inc. (Program guide on planning, policies, staff, transportation, readiness, precautions, records)

Thompson, M. *Recreation for the Homebound with Cerebral Palsy.* United Cerebral Palsy Associations, Inc. (A program guide to develop constructive activities for leisure time; bibliography and sample of records)

*Science Through Recreation.* Arlington, Va., Recreation Book Center, National Recreation and Park Association.

### Toys and Games

*Children Can Make It—Experiences in the World of Materials.* Washington, D.C., Association for Childhood Education, International.

Frantzen, J. *Toys . . . The Tools of Children.* Chicago, National Easter Seal Society for Crippled Children and Adults.

Herzoff, E. G. *It's Fun to Make Things from Scrap Materials.* New York, Dover Publications.

"Introduction to Homemade Games and Equipment." From *Recreation for the Mentally Retarded: A Handbook for Ward Personnel.* Atlanta, Southern Regional Education Board.

*Toy Book: Self-Help Toys to Make for Handicapped Children.* Indianapolis, Ind. Alpha Chi Omega National Headquarters.

### Modified Obstacle Course

Jones, M., Toczek, A. *Prenursery School Program for Children with CP.* New York, United Cerebral Palsy Associations, Inc. (A report by two physicians on a toddler-age program conducted at University of California at Los Angeles)

### University of Iowa Studies on Adapted Physical Education Programs

Bates, D. "The Effects of a Program of Balance Activities on Cerebral Palsied Children," Master's thesis, 1959.

Bok, F. "Evaluation of Improvement in Gait of Cerebral Palsied Children," Doctoral dissertation, 1956.

Healy, A. "A Comparison of Two Methods of Weight Training for Children with Spastic Type of Cerebral Palsy," Master's thesis, 1957.

McIntyre, M. "Recreation-time and Response-time Measurements in Children Afflicted with Cerebral Palsy," Master's thesis, 1961.

Meditch, C. "Effectiveness of Two Methods of Weight Training for Children with Athetoid Type of Cerebral Palsy," Master's thesis, 1961.

Soper, G. "A Study of Kinesthetic Sense in Children with Cerebral Palsy," Master's thesis, 1967.

Stoll, T. "The Effectiveness of a Special Program of Exercises on Eye-Hand Coordination in Children with Cerebral Palsy," Master's thesis, 1965.

### General References on Adapted Physical Education Programs

*Challenge.* (See under References: Guides for Recreational Activities)

Daniels, A. S. *Adapted Physical Education: Principles and Practice for Exceptional Students.* New York, Harper, 1954.

Fait, H. F. *Adapted Physical Education for Those with Physical and Mental Deviations and Low Physical Fitness.* Philadelphia, Saunders, 1960.

Marx, O. H. *Selected Bibliography for Physical Education and Recreation for Mentally Retarded and Physically Handicapped.* Iowa City, University Hospital School.

### Stuffed, Weighted Toy Animals

Auxter, D. "Basic movement experiences," Challenge 3:2, 1968.

Lounsberry, J. "Weight training for mentally retarded at primary level," Challenge 2:1, 1967.

### Music and Rhythm

"The Art and Music Programs at the Institute of Logopedics." Institute of Logopedics, Inc. (Reprint from *Cerebral Palsy Rev,* obtainable from Institute).

Barr, L. J. *Motion Songs for Tots.* National Recreation and Park Association. (Words, music, and suggested actions for 27 motion songs.)

Buttolph, E. *Music Is Motion.* National Recreation and Park Association. (Folk music and classical music for body movement through rhythms and songs.)

Knapp, I. *Teaching Aids for the Child's Unfoldment Through Music.* National Recreation and Park Association. (Rhythmics, toy orchestra, singing for preschoolers.)

"Music and Rhythm." *Recreation for the Mentally Retarded: A Handbook for Ward Personnel.* Southern Regional Education Board.

*Parent, Teacher and Younger Child.* National Recreation and Park Association.

"Records, Books, Rhythmic Instruments for Exceptional Children," Children's Music Center, Los Angeles, Calif. (Catalog)

*Records, Film Strips, and Instructional Materials.* Activity Records, Inc., Freeport, N.Y. (Finger games, singing action, games, and musical manners)

Saffran, R. *First Book of Creative Rhythms.* National Recreation and Park Association. (Music to accompany elementary motion.)

*Singing Games.* National Recreation and Park Association. (For youngsters age 5 to 7.)

Stuart, F. R., Ludlam, J. S. *Rhythmic Activities, Series I.* Minneapolis, Burgess Publishing Co. (Dances and games for young children, with simple scores or recommended recordings.)

# 12
# Children's Group Activities

Some suggestions for group activity for younger children were given in Chapter 11. As the child grows older, he will need a wider range of such activities, at least to the extent that he is physically able to participate in them. This chapter describes a number of types of group recreation in which such young people can take an active part.

## CAMPING

Camping affords the child or young adult a change from the routine of school and therapy and an opportunity for recreation and fun in a group setting. Some children are capable of fitting into camps organized for normal children. The local or state United Cerebral Palsy Association can suggest some of these.

Most cerebral palsied children will need camps that have adapted equipment, specialized staff members, and programs designed around their capabilities (Fig. 12-1).

## Sources for Information

American Camping Assoc.
Camp Fire Girls, Inc.
National Association for Retarded Children
National Recreation and Park Assoc.
United Cerebral Palsy Associations, Inc.
Kentucky Society for Crippled Children

## DAY CAMP EQUIPMENT

Equipment for day camping may be quite simple or very elaborate. It may be borrowed from the park, the public or private recreation center, loaned or donated by friends or families, or purchased by the agency. The United Cerebral Palsy Associations' Program Bulletin No. 11 gives the following suggestions for equipment and supplies needed to operate a day camp.

### Program Supplies

1. Baseballs and bats (senior or junior size)
2. Large balls and small balls
3. Bean bags
4. Paper bag puppets
5. Dolls, tables, dishes, chairs
6. Tear-out pictures

7. Blocks, plastic toys, and washable soft toys for free-play period
8. Checkers, pick-up sticks, and other table games for rainy days
9. Record player or piano
10. Rhythm orchestra instruments
11. Records, for enjoyment and for music and dance projects
12. Arts and crafts supplies

### General Equipment

1. Slide, see-saw, swings, and other appropriate playground equipment (these are usually available from the city or town recreation department)
2. Chairs and tables of the right height for different size people
3. Extra wheelchairs (which can be rented) to make some children more comfortable and others more mobile
4. Cots or blankets for rest period
5. First-aid equipment

### Storage Provision

Some provision must be made for storing equipment, particularly if the building is used by other

**FIG. 12-1.** Wheelchair baseball. The umpire calls the batter out. (Courtesy of United Cerebal Palsy of Nassau County, Roosevelt, N.Y.)

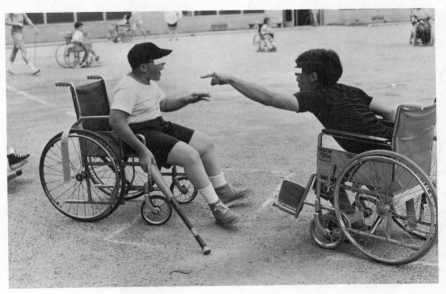

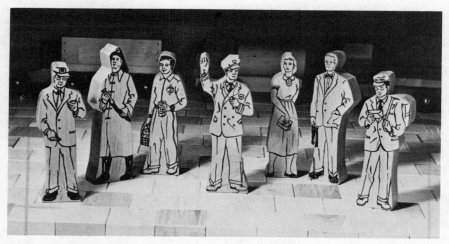

**FIG. 12-2.** Stand-up wooden figures used for Theme of the Week planned play. (Courtesy of Community Playthings, Rifton, N.Y.)

groups between times. Folding tables, chairs, and cots are often easiest to handle in this respect. It would be well also to look into the question of availability of a storage bin or large closet into which equipment can be placed when not in use.

## WEEK-LONG PLAY-LESSON PLAN

A planned play way is usable in residential and day care centers to acquaint youngsters with aspects of the world around them. One such lesson plan, suggested by George Garland of the Warren G. Murray Children's Center, Centralia, Ill., was used to acquaint retarded children with a community helper—the postman (Fig. 12-2). The plan is presented here to show how such an idea may be carried out.

### MONDAY

1. Self-expression—group-related experiences, receiving mail
2. Flannel board—samples of mail identification, such as stamps, addresses
3. Story—"Mr. Zip and the U.S. Mail"
4. Music—"Men Who Come to Our House"
5. Free play—Playskool postal boxes, playing postman with postal cards
6. Writing and drawing—writing letters or copying letters with paper and pencil; drawing pictures to send in a letter; writing or copying letters of names

### TUESDAY

1. Self-expression—color of postal box, mailman's uniform, and bag
2. Art—making and painting a large carton mailbox (the two chores are rotated among group members)
3. Free play—wood community helpers, postal boxes, "mail" (beads and blocks)
4. Story—reading and reviewing "Mr. Zip"

### WEDNESDAY

1. Self-expression—writing letters: how, why, where, and what to say
2. Art—collage made from stamps
3. Free play—no specific materials
4. Writing and drawing—writing letter (with help) or drawing pictures; mailing letters: folding, putting into envelope, addressing, and mailing in the postal boxes made in the group

### THURSDAY

Field trip to local post office

### FRIDAY

1. Self-expression—discussing trip
2. Campus mail travels—a walk from administration building to community building to a house to see how their letters travel to and from each child

## EVALUATION

After the week's program is complete, the adult leaders hold an evaluation session and group discussion concerning the week's experiences. Problems and difficulties of the experience are discussed and plans for the future theme and related activities are made.

## SWIMMING AND SWIMMING AIDS

Playing in the water and learning to swim can be one of the greatest pleasures from childhood on, and the therapeutic value of swimming has long been known. With proper precautions, many handicapped children are able to partake of such fun (Fig. 12-3). The use of pools is often offered free of charge to disabled youngsters by the YMCA, YWCA, and public and private schools, parks and playgrounds, and private clubs.

### Precautions

The precautions listed below are from Bulletin No. 10, *Swimming for the Cerebral Palsied,* of the United Cerebral Palsy Associations, Inc.

1. An adjustable canvas swim vest containing an air chamber which can be inflated to the degree desired has proved very satisfactory in providing buoyancy and correct body position, especially in severe cases.
2. A canvas-covered styrofoam adjustable belt is sometimes more beneficial when used on those whose arm movement is restricted.
3. Sometimes a combination of the items described above is most successful.
4. Inner tubes have proved to be only a toy. Kapok jackets are completely unsatisfactory.
5. Half-inflated plastic rings are satisfactory to hold onto for support while learning to kick the feet.
6. A heavy metal chair or folding metal ladder in the shallow water may be used as a diving aid to establish proper position for porpoise diving. However, safety precautions must be used so that the chairs will not be obstacles for other swimmers.

### KIDDIE BELT

The Kiddie Belt No. 4 is a belt with three floats (Fig. 12-4). For a tiny child, only two floats are needed; and for a huskier child an extra float can be added.

### Source

Ludington Plastics, Inc.

### SWIM-KWIK

This floater is made of two molded plastic parts with rubber straps (Fig. 12-5). The front or back plastic section can be removed as the swimmer gains proficiency.

### Source

Ocean Pool Supply Co.

### EXPANDED POLYETHYLENE

Expanded polyethylene can be used to make a satisfactory floater.

### Source

Dow Chemical Co.

### INNOVATION

Empty, clean, Clorox bottles, plastic, in ½- 1-gallon size with handles, with the caps screwed on tightly, make useful floaters. Youngsters who can hold onto the handles of these or similar bottles can strengthen their kicking in a more secure float position. The bottles can be used with or without float devices, depending upon the amount of support the child needs physically or emotionally.

## ADAPTED GAMES

Many kinds of games can be adapted for handicapped children. Some suggestions are given here, with their adaptations, that a group leader might not ordinarily think of as usable. With all such activities, however, advance planning and certain precautions are advisable. Jacob Schleichkorn of United Cerebral Palsy of New York State, prepared the following material for us.

### Precautions

1. Choose one adult to be in charge and responsible for planning the game.
2. Select a game suitable for age and mental level of the group.

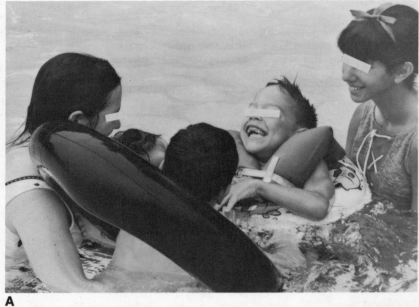

A

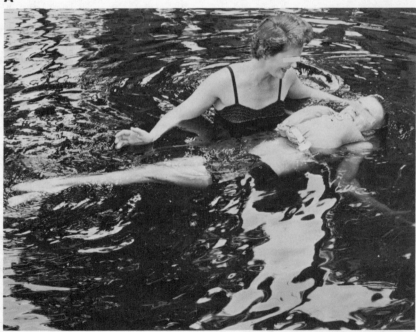

B

**FIG. 12-3.** The delights of learning to float and swim. (*A*) Young boy gets a thrill from being buoyed up in the water by his life-jacket. (*B*) Young adult learns to kick his feet while floating on his back. (Courtesy of United Cerebral Palsy of Nassau County, Roosevelt, N.Y. (*A*) and Tampa, Fla. (*B*)

3. Decide on the purpose and objectives of the activity.
4. Prepare a work plan.
5. Change the rules of the game to meet the physical ability of the group.
6. Keep it simple enough for children to understand and maintain interest.
7. Obtain all equipment before the period starts.
8. Have adequate assistance.
9. Select games that normal children play, as a basis of future communication.
10. Have everyone present, adults included, participate directly.
11. Avoid games that depend solely on competition of individuals for success.
12. Use games that bring some success to each player.
13. Allow sufficient time for all to participate.
14. Do not end the play abruptly; use a quiet game or song to end the play period.

## ADAPTATION OF "GIANT STEPS"

*Participants:* Ten moderately to severely disabled youngsters
*Purpose:* Practice in locomotion and speech; fun
*Assistants Needed:* Game director and one aide to help the individual child when necessary
*Special Equipment Needed:* None
*Adaptation:* One child on crutches with the adult near; one child who can propel his own wheelchair; one child who can push a child in a wheelchair; one child with a single cane; one child using two canes; four who are independent walkers
*Directions:* The group chooses a leader. The others stand about 25 feet away, facing the leader. As the leader calls out the number of steps, the player must say, "May I?" When given permission, the player goes the distance called. Any child may move forward secretly during the game, but if he is spotted by the leader, he must return to the starting line. The winner becomes the next leader.

## ADAPTATION OF BOWLING

*Participants:* Eight to 10 nonambulatory children, ages 5 to 9.
*Purpose:* Motion of the upper extremities; gross eye-hand coordination; fun
*Assistants Needed:* One director and one aide
*Special Equipment Needed:* A large basketball and several large, long wooden blocks

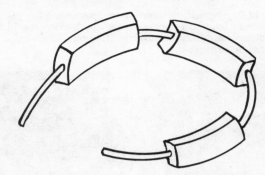

**FIG. 12-4.** Diagram of Kiddie Belt. Floats can be removed or added, as necessary. (Adapted from photograph of Ludington Plastics, Ludington, Mich.)

**FIG. 12-5.** Swim-Kwik. Plastic sections can be removed when the swimmer gains proficiency. (Adapted from photograph of Ocean Pool Supply, Huntington Station, N.Y.)

**FIG. 12-6.** Adapted bowling at a bowling alley. Boy in wheelchair learned to score so well by kicking the ball, he could join his family in bowling. (Courtesy of Chicago Day Camps, Chicago, Ill.)

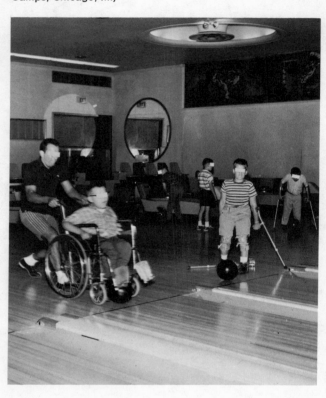

*Adaptations:* Ball large enough but not too heavy to enable children with poor grasp to manage

*Directions:* All players sit facing the wall with enough space between the seats and the wall for the game (5 to 15 feet). An adult sets up a number of blocks, staggering them so they knock one another over when hit by the ball. Three throws of the ball are given each child. The score is the number of blocks downed by the child or by the team.

## OTHER MODIFICATIONS OF BOWLING

It is possible for the handicapped child to enjoy the pleasures of a real bowling alley with adapted forms of playing. There are many ways of getting a ball down the alley: by sitting on the floor and pushing the ball; by support from one crutch while throwing the ball; or by holding the ball between the feet as the counselor runs the wheelchair up to the foul line for "kick-off" (Fig. 12-6).

## BOWLING AID

One adaptation for bowling is a chute which will send the ball down the alley. It consists of a metal frame and can be constructed (Fig. 12-9).

### Construction

1. Legs can be made of wood or metal.
2. Chute bottom is made of hardwood braced at top by hardwood blocks (*H*) and has cutouts (*K*) for attachment of sides, and holes (*L*) ½ inch in diameter.
3. Chute sides (*S*) made be made of ⅛-inch chip board or ½-inch plywood.
4. Chute rails (*J*) are of Bakelite or hardwood, with a notch (*G*) for ball stop.
5. Rubber (*A-E*) is applied at the base of the chute.
    Section *C-C* can also be purchased commercially.

### Sources for Information

Full instructions for constructing a metal frame bowling device may be obtained from:
Human Resources Center
United Cerebral Palsy of Denver, Inc.
United Cerebral Palsy of Northwestern Pennsylvania
For information about bowling as a competitive sport, as well as a spectator sport for adults contact the National Wheelchair Athletic Association.

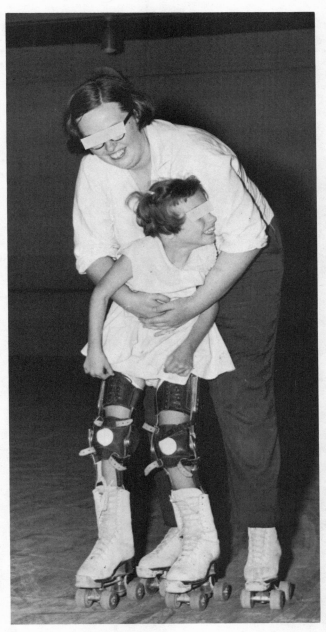

**FIG. 12-7.** Adult size roller-skating shoes fitted over braces. With the help of an aide, the little girl has an enjoyable sensory experience. (Courtesy of Chicago Day Camps, United Cerebral Palsy of Chicago)

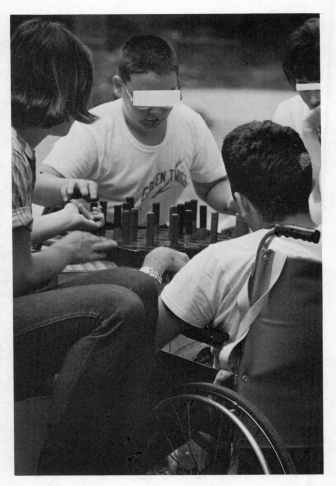

**FIG. 12-8.** Game of checkers, played with pegs in holes. Adaptation makes game easier for those with poor hand use. (Courtesy of United Cerebral Palsy of Nassau County, Roosevelt, N.Y.)

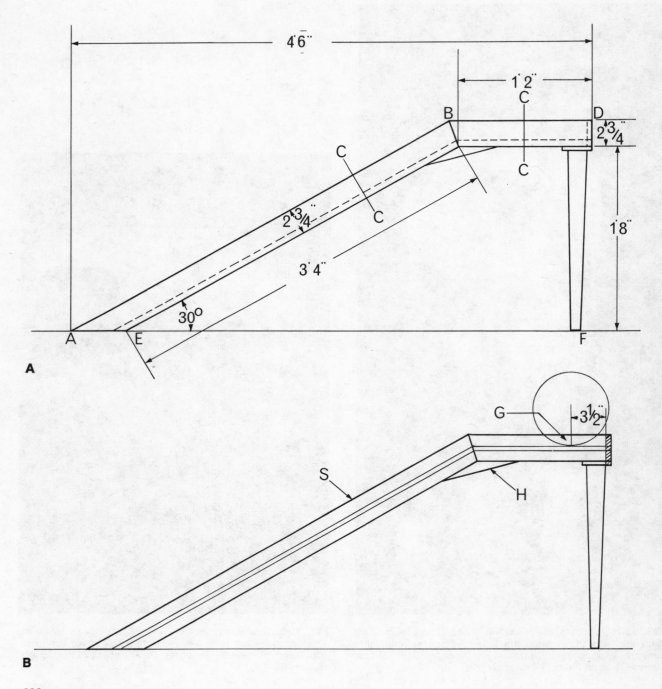

A

B

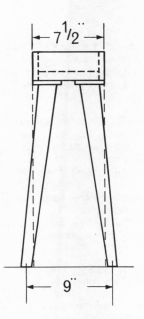

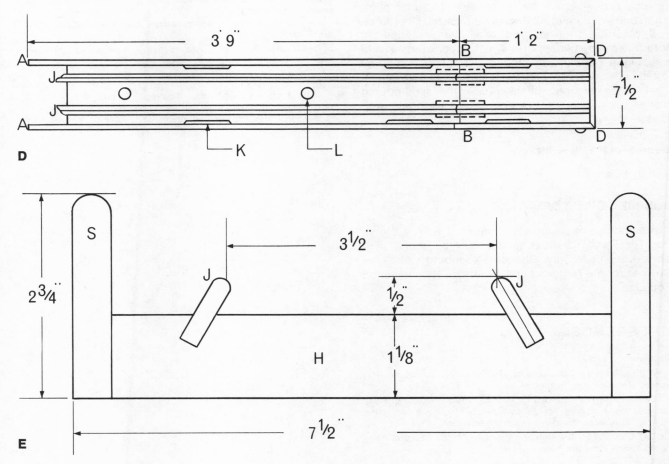

**FIG. 12-9.** Diagram for construction of bowling chute. (*A*) Side view showing dimensions: alley floor; bend in chute (B); chute (C—C); back edge where player stands (D); rubber mat on floor at bottom of chute. (*B*) Side view. (*C*) Rear view, showing dimensions. (*D*) Section C—C, showing supporting block, *H*; sides, *S*; (*E*) Top view of full length of chute, showing end resting on floor, *A*; rails, *J*; notches, *K*; bend in chute, *B*; and rear edge, *D*. (Courtesy of United Cerebal Palsy of North West Pennsylvania, Erie, Pa.)

## ADAPTATION OF SKATING

Some handicapped children can experience the fun of roller skating. Large shoes with wooden rollers attached can be applied over the child's braces (Fig. 12-7). With assistance the child can gain confidence and learn to achieve balance and, eventually, motion.

## ADAPTATIONS OF TABLE GAMES

It is possible for a child with cerebral palsy to play standard table games without letting aberrant motion knock the pieces out of place and disrupt the game. The process is often simple. A conventional game board can be mounted on wood. Holes may then be drilled into each space where movable pieces might rest during play. Pegs or dowel pieces which fit these holes can be painted the competitive colors of the original chips, checkers, or marbles (Fig. 12-8).

There are times when the game board is too small to allow enough space for the players to grip the pegs. Then construction of all items is indicated. One therapist, Beatrice Crowder, has used contact paper to form alternate squares of a checker board instead of painting a home-made model. She finds that large plastic checkers may be filled with sand to add weight. The side seams of the checkers are split, sand poured inside, and the checkers are sealed up again with tape.

### Source for Plastic Checkers

Rehab Aids

## SOURCE FOR INFORMATION

Adaptations of parcheesi, Chinese checkers, bingo, Peg-Tak-Toe, and other games may be found in a booklet compiled by Charlot Rosenberg: *Assistive Devices for the Handicapped,* American Rehabilitation Foundation.

# REFERENCES

### Camping

"A Bibliography on Camp Safety, Hygiene, and Sanitation," National Safety Council, Chicago, Ill.

"Camping Makes Life Worth Living," United Cerebral Palsy Associations, Inc., New York. (Documentary film, black and white, on how to organize and maintain a summer camp)

"Day Camping for the Cerebral Palsied," United Cerebral Palsy Associations, Inc., New York.

"Day Camping for Mentally Retarded," National Association for Retarded Children, Arlington, Texas.

"Directory of Camps for the Handicapped," American Camping Association, Martinsville, Ind. (Also available from the National Easter Seal Society for Crippled Children and Adults, Chicago, Ill.

"Guide for Day Camping," Camp Fire Girls, Inc., New York.

Schoenbohm, W. B. "Planning and Operating Facilities for Crippled Children," Springfield, Ill., Charles C. Thomas, 1962. (Chapter on planning a camp)

"Standards for Accredited Camps," American Camping Association.

"Camp Kysoc Manual" (Staff Manual), Kentucky Society for Crippled Children and Adults, Inc.

"Three Articles on Camping for the Handicapped" Rec Mag, National Recreation and Park Association.

### Swimming

*Seizures as Related to Waterfront and Playground Activities.* Epilepsy Society of Massachusetts. (Summary of precautions and emergency care)

"Swimming for the Cerebral Palsied," Program Bulletin 10, United Cerebral Palsy Associations, Inc. (Outlines how to set up a swimming program.)

"Swimming for the Handicapped," American National Red Cross, Washington, D.C.

"Techniques in Teaching Swimming to Handicapped," Henry Goodwin, West Chester State College. (Film)

### Bowling

Allen, R. "Experiments with Bowling," Challenge 3:1-4, Sept 1967. American Association for Health, Physical Education and Recreation. (Project on Recreation and Fitness for Mentally Retarded)

# 13
# Preteen and Young Adult Recreation

A wide variety of types of recreation are available for the preteen and young adult handicapped person: from Scouting to hobbies to ham radio operation to travel.

## SCOUTING

Scout troops are located in churches, YM or YW buildings, schools, institutions, day care centers, and recreation centers. Some regular troops have projects to serve disabled youngsters, some enroll youngsters with specific disabilities, and some limit enrollment to the capacity to follow the selected program.

At some institutions the troops are organized specifically for the residents, and in some instances the residents may be driven to the facilities of a local Scout troop. Troops meeting in day care centers or rehabilitation centers sometimes share space (Figs. 13-1 and 13-2). They may schedule a periodic social hour and special events with disabled youngsters, giving each the opportunity to share with the other and thus build for future citizenship.

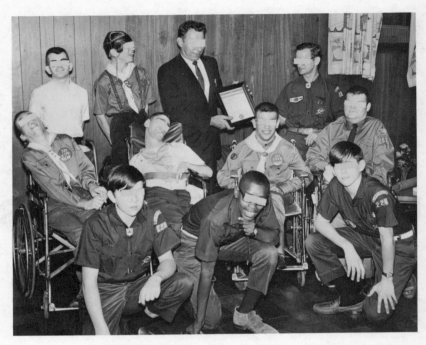

**FIG. 13-1.** Boy Scout Troop 521 for the cerebral palsied. The young men in the foreground are members of Troop 224 who assist the members of Troop 521. (Courtesy of United Cerebral Palsy Association of Philadelphia and vicinity)

**FIG. 13-2.** Girl Scout Troop 1116 for the cerebral palsied. (Courtesy of United Cerebral Palsy Association of Philadelphia and vicinity)

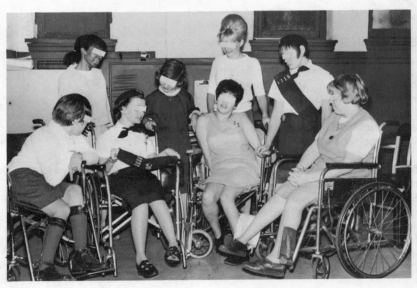

### Table 13-1. SCOUTING UNITS FOR BOYS WITH CEREBRAL PALSY

| Unit | Sponsor |
|---|---|
| Troop #682 | Mid-State Cerebral Palsy Center<br>125 State Street, Augusta, Me. 04330 |
| Troop #360<br>Pack #3360 | Cerebral Palsy of Essex County and<br>    West Hudson<br>7 Sanford Avenue, Belleville, N.J. 07109 |
| Pack #3112 | Cerebral Palsy Center<br>28 Baldwin Street, Johnson City, N.Y. 13790 |
| Post #2995 | Syracuse Cerebral Palsy Center<br>W. Seneca Tpk., Syracuse, N.Y. 13207 |
| Troop #350<br>Post #2350 | United Cerebral Palsy of Nassau County<br>380 Washington, Roosevelt, N.Y. 11575 |
| Troop #90 | Rehabilitation Program, Inc.<br>North Road, Poughkeepsie, N.Y. 12601 |
| Troop #521 | United Cerebral Palsy Assn.<br>2545 N. Broad Street,<br>Philadelphia, Pa. 19132 |
| Troop #330<br>Post #2330 | United Cerebral Palsy of Washington, D.C.<br>1330 Massachusetts Avenue, N.W.<br>Washington, D.C. 20005 |
| Troop #301<br>Troop #471<br>Pack #3301 | Cerebral Palsy School & DAV Chapter 89<br>1520 Baxter Avenue, Louisville, Ky. 40205 |
| Troop #123<br>Pack #3123 | United Cerebral Palsy Assn.<br>112 Perry Drive, N.W., Canton, Ohio 44708 |
| Troop #916<br>Post #2916<br>Pack #3916 | Butler County Assn. of Cerebral Palsy &<br>    Mentally Retarded Children<br>323 N. 3rd Street, Hamilton, Ohio 45011 |
| Troop #450<br>Pack #3006 | Cerebral Palsy Center<br>Pensacola, Fla. 32504 |
| Troop #1072<br>Pack #3222 | Greensboro Cerebral Palsy &<br>    Orthopedic School<br>1508 Gatewood Drive<br>Greensboro, N.C. 27405 |
| Troop #599 | United Cerebral Palsy Center<br>2727 Columbine Street, Denver, Colo. 80205 |
| Post #2202 | United Cerebral Palsy of Oklahoma City<br>3701 S. 29th, Oklahoma City, Okla. 73119 |
| Pack #3827 | Cerebral Palsy Center<br>2000 N.E. 150th St., Seattle, Wash. 98155 |
| Troop #105<br>Pack #3105 | West Contra Costa Cerebral Palsy Society<br>El Cerrito, Calif. 94530 |

Camps may be a good place to initiate the disabled youngster into the skills and group behavior that will help him to team up with troops in winter.

## SCOUTING UNITS FOR THE DISABLED

Scouting units for disabled boys and girls exist all over the United States. The listing given in Table 13-1 may serve as a source of information concerning experience, adaptations, and precautions for leaders wishing to organize such troops.

### Scouting and Camp Fire Headquarters

Boy Scouts of America
Girl Scouts of the U.S.A.
Camp Fire Girls, Inc.

## EDUCATIONAL HOBBIES

Hobbies can be as important as jobs. Everyone needs a few hobbies, and those that the handicapped person may enjoy are legion—pets, nature, spectator sports, art, weather—the list goes on. Some brief suggestions are given here, with sources of information about them. Do remember that your local public library is an excellent source to supplement these.

### BIRDS

The National Audubon Society is a central resource for bird lovers. For those interested in observing the migrations of wild birds, the government has issued a useful pamphlet on why they do so, when, the dangers they encounter, etc.

### Source

Office of Conservation Education, Bureau of Sport Fisheries & Wildlife (Pamphlet No. 8: *The Migration of Birds*)

### HOME ECONOMICS

Sewing, embroidery, knitting, crocheting, etc., can be enjoyable hobbies for those with good hand use and may be profitable, too.

### Source

Johnson's Wax (Pamphlet of low-budget ideas on *Easy-To-Make Gifts*).

### LANGUAGE ARTS

Becoming familiar with the lingo of a particular occupation can be fun and a means of communicating with new people.

### Source

The Propeller Club of the United States (Folder on how to correspond with a ship's captain: *Adopt-a-Ship Plan*).

### MUSIC

Singing or learning to play an instrument, from a recorder on up; becoming familiar with great operas or great composers; getting to know all about jazz—the field of music has a wide range of hobbies to offer.

### Source

Stephen Foster Memorial (A book of Stephen Foster's songs, including words and music, is available; it is valuable to any teacher who plays the piano).

### BASEBALL

With the popularity of baseball and other sports of TV, getting to know about the rules of the game and its stars can be a hobby for the whole family.

### Source

Hillerich and Bradsby Co., Inc. (Baseball rule book).

### RAILROADS

Getting to know how the railroad developed in the United States and the impact on national growth can be fascinating.

### Source

Association of American Railroads

### "NATURE" MAGAZINE

Learning about nature, ecology and joining naturalists through pictures and reports of their projects can be rewarding.

### Source

American Museum of Natural History, Education Division

### NATIONAL AND STATE PARKS

Many a pleasant trip—real or imaginary—can be planned if one has a good knowledge about the various facilities in the country and what they have to offer.

### Source

Phillips Petroleum Co., Editorial Division (*Guide to Your National Forests, Parks, Monuments and Historic Sites*, listed by states)

### WEATHER

A hobbyist weather forecaster could be a very popular person.

### Source

Scott, Foresman and Co. (Chart, 21 by 25 inches, No. A2440, "What Can We Learn from a Weather Record?" for primary teachers. Specific items only available as long as supply lasts; then substitutions will be made).

## HOBBIES THROUGH CORRESPONDENCE

Hobbies can often be shared with others through another hobby—pen pals. It is also a good way to develop *new* hobbies.

*Rehabilitation Gazette,* a periodical of information for and by severely disabled persons, is an excellent means of sharing your hobby with others. There are over 1,400 persons on the *Gazette's* mailing list. Seventy-three percent are between 20 and 39 years of age: 38 percent have completed college, 40 percent can write, and 38 percent can type in spite of their disabilities.

Contacts can also be made through special-interest groups.

### Sources for Information

Accent Pen Pals
Association of Handicapped Artists
*Rehabilitation Gazette* Catalog of Handicapped Hams (radio ham operators).
Correspondence League of America for Chess
Homebound Book Service (mailing of books to the handicapped; free catalog).
Pen Pals. *Rehabilitation Gazette* will furnish a free ad if writer will send name, address, age, hobbies, languages that he writes. The ad should be brief but have enough information to attract a response from readers with similar interests.
*Rehabilitation Gazette* There are no subscriptions, but a tax-deductible donation is welcome from both the disabled and the nondisabled.

### WRITING

For those engaged in writing stories or articles, it is possible to find out which publishers are interested in having such material submitted and the types of material they are likely to accept.

### Sources for Information

The Writer Inc.
Writers' Digest

### TAPE CLUBS

Those who own tape recorders can make contacts with others having the same interests through several organizations. Most of these clubs are run by other disabled individuals on a shoestring budget, so it is advisable to send a self-addressed, stamped envelope for information.

### Sources for Information

*Rehabilitation Gazette* Clubless Tape Correspondence (For memo and information about the *Tape Recording Magazine,* send name, address, age, kind of tape recorder owned, speed, and number of tracks, subjects on which "tapesponding" is desired, and language spoken.)
The Voicespondence Club

## HAM RADIO OPERATION

Ham radio operating is an activity which can be carried on without leaving the house, and although good speech is helpful, it is not absolutely necessary.

In the "CP News," published by United Cerebral Palsy of Philadelphia and vicinity, was the story of R.C., who became a ham operator. He was always interested in radio, and when someone gave him a "Citizen's Band Transmitter" radio several years ago, he became an active operator (Fig. 13-3). This made it possible for him to communicate with other operators in the Philadelphia area. Through this he learned how to place calls properly, methods of receiving, and something about circuitry.

Then he studied for a written exam which included Morse code, radio law, circuitry, and fundamentals of electronics. He passed the test and received his amateur radio license. This permitted him to operate on over four million frequencies and to communicate around the world. He now uses a "transceiver," through which he can use voice, Morse code, and teletype. He can receive emergency messages through Eastern Pennsylvania Emergency Phone and Traffic Network, and relay these by phone—a public service performed by ham operators.

### Pointers

A good band transmitter radio may be bought second hand for about $50. Second-hand transceivers have been purchased by hams for about $200.

## TRAVELING

Physical disability need not deter those who wish to travel if they are able to get about at home. (Fig. 13-4). A number of tours and travel guides are available which will help the handicapped person plan and enjoy a trip.

See the special travel issue of *Rehabilitation Gazette* (Spring 1965) for details on travel tips and for interesting reports of trips taken by disabled persons.

The May–June 1967 issue of *Rehabilitation Record* notes that Holiday Inns have new construction plans calling for two rooms out of every 100 to be fully equipped for handicapped travelers: wide parking spaces close to rooms, rooms close to restaurants, bathroom doors widened, and ramps constructed where needed. Perhaps this will establish a good precedent for others to follow.

### Sources for Information on Tours

Mrs. Dorothy S. Axsom, Sponsor. Tours for the Handicapped, Handy-Cap Horizons. (Tours to New York, Washington, D.C., and Hollywood, Miami, and Chicago).

Miss Betty Hoffman, Evergreen Travel Service

### Sources for Travel Guides

British Red Cross Society. Directory of Holidays for the Handicapped in Britain. Places to stay, care available, age groups, prices and nearby entertainment.

Travelodge Corp. Directory of Travelodges and Supplement. Units designed for wheelchair use.

The President's Committee on Employment of the Handicapped. Guide to the National Parks and Monuments for Handicapped Tourists. A directory of over 200 tourist attractions in the national park system, telling whether museums, visitor centers, and concession stands are accessible to persons with ambulatory limitations. Forewarns about steps, narrow doorways, inaccessible toilets, or other architectural barriers.

Guide to Washington for the Handicapped. Society for Crippled Children, Guides for the Handicapped. An up-to-date list of 32 cities. Architectural Barriers Project, National Easter Seal Society for Crippled Children and Adults.

Robert L. Webb, Editor, Paraplegia News. Wheelchair Travel Guide

Paralyzed Veterans of America. Where the Turning Wheels Stop.

## EXCLUSIVELY AIR TRAVEL

Handicapped persons who may confront difficulties in boarding aircraft or in otherwise traveling by means of the nation's airways will find help at their fingertips in a new publication released by the National Easter Seal Society for Crippled Children and Adults.

*Airline Transportation for the Handicapped and Disabled,* a booklet prepared by rehabilitation specialist Stanley G. Hogsett, surveys the policies and pro-

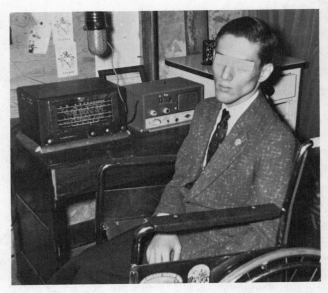

**FIG. 13-3.** Ham radio operation as an adult hobby for the cerebral palsied. R. C., of Philadelphia, is now a full-fledged ham operator. (Courtesy of United Cerebral Palsy Association of Philadelphia and vicinity)

**FIG. 13-4.** Disability no bar to travel. A handicapped traveler disembarks from a flight. (Courtesy of Audio Visual Unit, Research Utilization Branch, SRS-HEW)

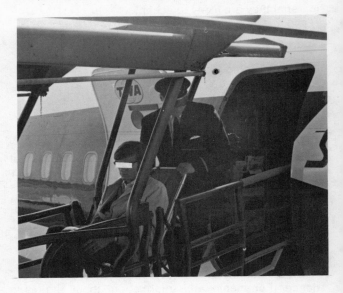

cedures established by 22 domestic airlines as well as by the Air Transport Association of America and the Civil Aeronautics Board in handling handicapped passengers.

The report presents the first comprehensive picture of its kind, offering assurance that with careful planning even those with severe disabilities can surmount special problems and enjoy the convenience and pleasure of air travel.

Information the author has compiled holds the resource help needed by all persons who accompany a disabled individual or assist with his flight plans, including physicians who must make decisions regarding fitness for air travel of patients seeking this advice.

Included in *Airline Transportation for the Handicapped and Disabled* are:

—medical criteria considered by airlines and physical and mental conditions that might be contradictory to airline travel or require special planning.

—services offered to handicapped and disabled passengers by individual airlines, and

—requirements set generally as well as specifically for persons with limited mobility and those who use oxygen or who are blind, pregnant, mentally retarded or mentally ill, or handicapped by other conditions.

**Source**

National Easter Seal Society for Crippled Children and Adults, the report (Publications #E-47) is available at $1.25 a copy.

# REFERENCES

**Scouting**

*Handicapped Girls and Girl Scouting: Guide for Leaders.* New York, Girl Scouts of the USA, 1968.

*Scouting for the Mentally Retarded.* New Brunswick, N.J.,Boy Scouts of America, 1966.

*These Are Our Brothers.* Geneva, Switzerland, Boy Scouts World Bureau. (A guide to scouting with the handicapped)

# SOURCES FOR
# AIDS AND INFORMATION

**ACCENT PEN PALS**
P.O. Box 726
BLOOMINGTON, ILL.
61701

**ACTIVITY RECORDS, INC.**
FREEPORT, N.Y.
11520

**ADAPTIVE CREEPERS**
P.O. Box 26
PLYMOUTH, MICH.
48170

**ADJUSTA-CHAIR CO.**
12704 Brumley Drive
BRIDGETON, MO.
63044

**ADULTRIKE MANUFACTURING CO.**
Division of Custom Cycle
12209 Grand Ave.
EL MIRAGE, ARIZ.
85335

**ALLIED BODY WORKS, INC.**
3922 Seventh St. South
SEATTLE, WASH.
98146

**ALPHA CHI OMEGA NATIONAL HEADQUARTERS**
3445 N. Washington Blvd.
INDIANAPOLIS, IND.
46205

**AMERICAN ASSOCIATION FOR HEALTH, PHYSICAL EDUCATION AND RECREATION**
1201 Sixteenth St., N.W.
WASHINGTON, D.C.
20036

**AMERICAN CAMPING ASSOC.**
Bradford Woods
MARTINSVILLE, IND.
46151

**AMERICAN FOUNDATION FOR THE BLIND**
15 W. Sixteenth St.
NEW YORK, N.Y.
10011

**AMERICAN GUIDANCE SERVICE, INC.**
Publishers Bldg.
CIRCLE PINES, MINN.
55014

**AMERICAN HOSPITAL SUPPLY**
Division of American Hospital Supply Corp.
1450 Waukegan Road
McGAW PARK, ILL.
60085

**THE AMERICAN HUMANE ASSOC.**
P.O. Box 1226
DENVER, COLO.
80201

**AMERICAN LEGION**
Americanism Division
P.O. Box 1055
INDIANAPOLIS, IND.
46206

**AMERICAN NATIONAL RED CROSS**
17 and D Sts. N.W.
WASHINGTON, D.C.
20006

**AMERICAN OCCUPATIONAL THERAPY ASSOC.**
251 Park Ave. South
NEW YORK, N.Y.
10010

**AMERICAN REHABILITATION FOUNDATION**
1800 Chicago Ave.
MINNEAPOLIS, MINN.
55404

**AMERICAN SEATING CO.**
GRAND RAPIDS, MICH.
49504

**AMERICAN WHEELCHAIR**
5500 Muddy Creek Road
CINCINNATI, OHIO
45238
   also
LODOGA, IND.
47954

**AMPUTEE SHOE AND GLOVE EXCHANGE**
Dr. and Mrs. Richard E. Wainerdi
1115 Langford Drive
COLLEGE STATION, TEX.
77840

**APPLETON-CENTURY-CROFTS**
440 Park Ave. South
NEW YORK, N.Y.
10016

**ASSOCIATE COMMITTEE ON
THE NATIONAL BUILDING CODE**
National Research Council of Canada
OTTAWA, ONTARIO
CANADA
KLA OR 6

**ASSOCIATION OF AMERICAN RAILROADS**
Public Relations Department
American Railroads Building
WASHINGTON, D.C.
20036

**ASSOCIATION FOR CHILDHOOD
EDUCATION INTERNATIONAL**
3615 Wisconsin Ave., N.W.
Washington, D.C.
20016

**ASSOCIATION OF HANDICAPPED ARTISTS, INC.**
1134 Rand Building
BUFFALO, N.Y.
14203

**ASSOCIATION OF HOSPITAL AND
INSTITUTIONAL LIBRARIES**
50 East Huron St.
CHICAGO, ILL.
60611

**AUDIO BOOK CO.**
301 Pasadena Ave.
SOUTH PASADENA, CALIF.
91030

**B & L ENGINEERING**
9126 East Firestone Blvd., Bldg. R.
DOWNEY, CALIF.
90241

**BACHARACH-RASIN**
Gleneagles Court
TOWSON, MD.
21204

**BOB L. BEASLEY**
Physical Education Department
University of Southern Florida
TAMPA, FLA.
33620

**BELL & HOWELL CO.**
Audio-Visual Products Division
7100 McCormick Road
CHICAGO, ILL.
60645

**CHANNING L. BETE CO., INC.**
45 Federal St.
GREENFIELD, MASS.
01301

**DELORES A. BLACK**
Women's Physical Education and Recreation
 Department
Bowling Green State University
BOWLING GREEN, OHIO
43403

**J. J. BLOCK**
Aids for the Handicapped
1111 W. Argyle
CHICAGO, ILL.
60640

**BOOK-LAB, INC.**
1449 37 St.
BROOKLYN, N.Y.
11218

**BOY SCOUTS OF AMERICA**
NEW BRUNSWICK, N.J.
08902

**BOY SCOUTS WORLD BUREAU**
Case Postale 78
1211 Geneva 4
SWITZERLAND

**THE BRITISH RED CROSS SOCIETY**
9 Grosvenor Crescent
LONDON, SWIX 7EJ
England

**BUREAU OF OUTDOOR RECREATION**
U.S. Department of the Interior
WASHINGTON, D.C.
20240

**BUSH ELECTRIC CO.**
1245 Folsom St.
SAN FRANCISCO, CALIF.
94103

**CAEDMON RECORDS, INC.**
505 Eighth Ave.
NEW YORK, N.Y.
10018

**CAMP FIRE GIRLS, INC.**
1740 Broadway
NEW YORK, N.Y.
10019

**CATALOG OF FREE TEACHING MATERIALS**
P.O. Box 1075
VENTURA, CALIF.
93001

**CHECKER MOTOR SALES CORP.**
2016 N. Pitcher
KALAMAZOO, MICH.
49007

**CHILDCRAFT EDUCATION CORP.**
964 Third Ave.
NEW YORK, N.Y.
10022
    also
150 East 58 St.
NEW YORK, N.Y.
10022

**CHILDREN'S HOUSE MAGAZINE**
P.O. Box 111
CALDWELL, N.J.
07006

**CHILDREN'S MUSIC CENTER**
5373 W. Pico Blvd.
LOS ANGELES, CALIF.
90019

**CHILDREN TODAY**
Superintendent of Documents
U.S. Government Printing Office
WASHINGTON, D.C.
20402

**CLEO LIVING AIDS**
3957 Mayfield Road
CLEVELAND, OHIO
44121

**CLOTHING RESEARCH AND
DEVELOPMENT FOUNDATION**
48 E. 66 St.
NEW YORK, N.Y.
10021

**COLSON CO.**
39 S. Lasalle St.
CHICAGO, ILL.
60603

**COMMUNITY PLAYTHINGS**
RIFTON, N.Y.
12471

**CONSTRUCTIVE PLAYTHINGS**
1040 E. 85 St.
KANSAS CITY, MO.
64131

**THE CONTINENTAL PRESS, INC.**
ELIZABETHTOWN, PA.
17022

**COPPERLOY CORP.**
8901 East Pleasant Valley Road
CLEVELAND, OHIO
44131

**CORRESPONDENCE CHESS LEAGUE OF AMERICA**
P.O. Box 4157
CINCINNATI, OHIO
45204

**CREATIVE PLAYTHINGS**
PRINCETON, N.J.
08540

**CURTIS CIRCULATION CO.**
841 Chestnut St.
PHILADELPHIA, PA.
19105

**DEEMER-HOWARD ASSOCIATES, INC.**
P.O. Box 15129
LAS VEGAS, NEV.
89114

**D. C. DENISON ORTHOPAEDIC APPLIANCE CORP.**
220 W. 28 St.
BALTIMORE, MD.
21211

**DENTAL GUIDANCE COUNCIL
FOR CEREBRAL PALSY**
c/o United Cerebral Palsy Association of
   New York City
339 East 44 St.
NEW YORK, N.Y.
10016

**DEVELOPMENTAL LEARNING MATERIALS**
7440 N. Natchez Ave.
NILES, ILL.
60648

**DISTRICT OF COLUMBIA SOCIETY
FOR CRIPPLED CHILDREN, INC.**
2800-13 St., N.W.
WASHINGTON, D.C.
20009

**DIVISION FOR THE BLIND AND
PHYSICALLY HANDICAPPED**
Library of Congress
WASHINGTON, D.C.
20542

**DOVER CORPORATION/ELEVATOR DIVISION**
P.O. Box 2177
MEMPHIS, TENN.
38102

**DOW CHEMICAL CO.**
45 Rockefeller Plaza
NEW YORK, N.Y.
10020

**EATON E-Z BATH CO.**
P.O. Box 712
GARDEN CITY, KANS.
67846

**THE EDMUND SCIENTIFIC CO.**
555 Edscorp Bldg.
BARRINGTON, N.J.
08007

**EDUCATIONAL RESEARCH SERVICES, INC.**
7 Holland Ave.
WHITE PLAINS, N.Y.
10603

**EDUCATIONAL TEACHING AIDS**
159 W. Kinzie St.
CHICAGO, ILL.
60610

**EDUCATIONAL TESTING SERVICE**
Box 592
PRINCETON, N.J.
08540

**EDU KAID OF RIDGEWOOD**
RIDGEWOOD, N.J.
07450

**ENRICHMENT RECORDS**
50 West 44 St.
NEW YORK, N.Y.
10036

**EPILEPSY SOCIETY OF MASSACHUSETTS**
140 Boylston St.
BOSTON, MASS.
02116

**EVEREST & JENNINGS, INC.**
1803 Pontius Ave.
LOS ANGELES, CALIF.
90025
    also
165 Spring St.
MURRAY HILL, N.J.
07971

**EXECUTONE, INC.**
Special Education Division
J. A. Richards, Educational Director
47-37 Austell Place
LONG ISLAND CITY, N.Y.
11101

**FAIRWAY KING, INC.**
3 E. Main
OKLAHOMA CITY, OKLA.
73104

**FEDERATION OF THE HANDICAPPED**
211 W. 14 St.
NEW YORK, N.Y.
10011

**FOLKWAY RECORDS**
701 Seventh Ave.
NEW YORK, N.Y.
10036

**FOLLETT PUBLISHING CO.**
1010 West Washington Blvd.
CHICAGO, ILL.
60607

**FORD MOTOR CO.**
Medical Director, World Headquarters
Room 299
The American Road
DEARBORN, MICH.
48121

**FRANKLIN BODY & EQUIPMENT CORP.**
1042 Dean St.
BROOKLYN, N.Y.
11238

**MARIANNE FROSTIG CENTER
OF EDUCATIONAL THERAPY**
5981 Venice Blvd.
LOS ANGELES, CALIF.
90034

**GENERAL LEARNING CORP.**
The Judy Co.
250 James St.
MORRISTOWN, N.J.
07960

**GIRL SCOUTS OF THE U.S.A.**
830 Third Ave.
NEW YORK, N.Y.
10022

**GOBBY MANUFACTURING, INC.**
P.O. Box 274
6645 N. 58 Ave.
GLENDALE, ARIZ.
85301

**HENRY GOODWIN**
West Chester State College
School of Physical Education
WEST CHESTER, PA.
19380

**GREWE & SCHULTE-DERNE**
4628 Lunen/Westf
DERNER STRASSE 136
GERMANY

**HANDI-RAMP, INC.**
904 Countryside Highway
MUNDELEIN, ILL.
60060

**HANDY CAP HORIZONS**
Mrs. Dorothy S. Axsom, Sponsor
Tours for the Handicapped
3250 East Loretta Drive
INDIANAPOLIS, IND.
46227

**HAUSMANN INDUSTRIES, INC.**
130 Union St.
NORTHVALE, N.J.
07647

**HERITAGE HOUSE**
CLADDS FORD, PA.
19317

**HIGHLAND VIEW HOSPITAL**
3901 Ireland Drive
CLEVELAND, OHIO
44122

**HILLERICH AND BRADSBY CO., INC.**
P.O. Box 506
LOUISVILLE, KY.
40201

**MRS. BETTY J. HOFFMAN**
Evergreen Travel Service, Inc.
19429 44 Ave. W.
LYNNWOOD, WASH.
98036

**HOGG CHAIR CO.**
7722 S. Chicago
CHICAGO, ILL.
60619

**HOMEBOUND BOOK SERVICE**
Box 354
FAIR LAWN, N.J.
07410

**TED HOYER & COMPANY, INC.**
2222 Minnesota St.
OSHKOSH, WISC.
54901

**THE HUFFMAN MANUFACTURING CO.**
P.O. Box 1204
DAYTON, OHIO
45401

**HUMAN RESOURCES CENTER**
I.U. Willets Road
ALBERTSON, N.Y.
11507

**ICTA INFORMATION CENTRE**
Fack
S-161 03 Bromma 3
SWEDEN

**IDEAL SCHOOL SUPPLY CO.**
11000 S. Lavergne Ave.
OAK LAWN, ILL.
60453

**IDEAL TOY CORP.**
4135 S. Pulaski
CHICAGO, ILL.
60632

**INCLINATOR CO. OF AMERICA**
2200 Paxton St.
P.O. Box 1557
HARRISBURG, PA.
17105

**INCLINATOR-ELEVETTE CO. OF NEW YORK, INC.**
1213 Teaneck Road
TEANECK, N.J.
07666

**INSTITUTE OF LOGOPEDICS, INC.**
2400 Jardine Drive
WICHITA, KANS.
67219

**INVACARE CORP.**
443 Oberlin Road
ELYRIA, OHIO
44035

**A. JOHNSON AND A. WOLFE**
United Cerebral Palsy, Nursery School
University of California
LOS ANGELES, CALIF.
90024

**JOHNSON'S WAX**
Consumer Education Center
P.O. Box 567—Dept. MH
14 and Franklin Sts.
RACINE, WISC.
53403

**KEEFE AND KEEFE**
429 East 75 St.
NEW YORK, N.Y.
10021

**THE KENDALL CO.**
Hospital Products Division
309 West Jackson Blvd.
CHICAGO, ILL.
60606

**KENNER PRODUCTS**
912 Sycamore St.
CINCINNATI, OHIO
45202

**KENTUCKY SOCIETY FOR CRIPPLED CHILDREN AND ADULTS, INC.**
233 East Broadway
LOUISVILLE, KY.
40202

**LAMINEX, INC.**
5262 Independence St.
MAPLE PLAIN, MINN.
55359

**LARGE TYPE WEEKLY**
New York Times
229 W. 43 St.
NEW YORK, N.Y.
10036

**LISTENING LIBRARY, INC.**
1 Park Ave.
OLD GREENWICH, CONN.
06870

**LUDINGTON PLASTICS, INC.**
P.O. Box 176
LUDINGTON, MICH.
49431

**LUMEX, INC.**
100 Spence St.
BAY SHORE, N.Y.
11706

**MAFEX ASSOCIATES, INC.**
111 Barron Ave.
JOHNSTOWN, PA.
15906

**MEDI, INC.**
Box 325
27 Maple Ave.
HOLBROOK, MASS.
02343

**MEYRA WHEELCHAIRS FACTORY**
Wilhelm Meyer, Director
4973 VLOTHO/Weser
P.O. Box 103
GERMANY

**ARTHUR G. MILLER**
School of Education
Boston University
BOSTON, MASS.
02215

**G. E. MILLER, INC.**
484 S. Broadway
YONKERS, N.Y.
10705

**MINIBUS, INC.**
PICO RIVERA, CALIF.
90660

**MOONWALKER OF SPACE GENERAL CO.**
9200 East Flair Drive
EL MONTE, CALIF.
91731

**WARREN G. MURRAY CHILDREN'S CENTER**
1717 West Broadway
CENTRALIA, ILL.
62801

**NATIONAL ASSOCIATION
FOR RETARDED CHILDREN**
2709 Avenue E. East
ARLINGTON, TEX.
76011

**NATIONAL ASSOCIATION
FOR VISUALLY HANDICAPPED**
3201 Balboa St.
SAN FRANCISCO, CALIF.
94121

**NATIONAL AUDUBON SOCIETY**
Educational Services Department
950 Third Ave.
NEW YORK, N.Y.
10022

**NATIONAL EASTER SEAL SOCIETY
FOR CRIPPLED CHILDREN AND ADULTS**
2023 W. Odgen Ave.
CHICAGO, ILL.
60612

**NATIONAL HOME STUDY COUNCIL**
1601 18 St., N.W.
WASHINGTON, D.C.
20009

**NATIONAL RECREATION AND PARK ASSOC.**
1601 North Kent St.—11 Floor
ARLINGTON, VA.
22209

**NATIONAL SAFETY COUNCIL**
425 N. Michigan Ave.
CHICAGO, ILL.
60611

**NATIONAL SOCIETY FOR THE
PREVENTION OF BLINDNESS, INC.**
79 Madison Ave.
NEW YORK, N.Y.
10016

**NATIONAL UIVERSITY EXTENSION ASSOC.**
One Dupont Circle, Suite 360
WASHINGTON, D.C.
20036

**NATIONAL WHEELCHAIR ATHLETIC ASSOC.**
40-24 62 St.
WOODSIDE, N.Y.
11377

**"NATURE" MAGAZINE**
Education Department
American Museum of National History
79 St. at Central Park West
NEW YORK, N.Y.
10025

**NELSON ENTERPRISES**
4921 Gary St.
SAN DIEGO, CALIF.
92115

**NEW READERS PRESS**
Division of Lauback Literacy, Inc.
Box 131, University Station
SYRACUSE, N.Y.
13210

**NEW YORK STATE DEPARTMENT
OF MENTAL HYGIENE**
Office of Community Facilities Planning
44 Holland Ave.
ALBANY, N.Y.
12208

**NEW YORK STATE EDUCATION DEPARTMENT**
Bureau for Physically Handicapped Children
55 Elk St.
ALBANY, N.Y.
12224

**NEW YORK UNIVERSITY MEDICAL CENTER**
Institute of Rehabilitation Medicine
400 East 34 St.
NEW YORK, N.Y.
10016

**NISSEN CORP.**
930 27 Ave., S.W.
CEDAR RAPIDS, IOWA
52406

**NOAIR MANUFACTURING CO.**
Box 187
FARMINGDALE, N.Y.
11735

**OCEAN POOL SUPPLY CO.**
Stepar Place
HUNTINGTON STATION, N.Y.
11746

**OFFICE OF CONSERVATION EDUCATION,
PUBLICATIONS UNIT**
Bureau of Sport Fisheries & Wildlife
Room 617
1717 H St., N.W.
WASHINGTON, D.C.
20240

**OFFICIAL GUIDE TO CATHOLIC
EDUCATIONAL INSTITUTIONS**
200 Sunrise Highway
ROCKVILLE CENTRE, L.I., N.Y.
11570

**WALTER L. OLSEN**
Department of Special Education
University of Arizona
TUCSON, ARIZ.
85717

**ORTHOPEDIC EQUIPMENT CO.**
BOURBON, IND.
46504

**ORTHOPEDIC SERVICES OF RHODE ISLAND**
340 Broad St.
PROVIDENCE, R.I.
02907

**ORTHOPEDIC SUPPLIES CO.**
9126 E. Firestone Blvd.
DOWNEY, CALIF.
90241

**ORTOPEDIA GMBH**
23 Kiel 14
SALZREDDER, 3
GERMANY

**PARALYZED VETERANS OF AMERICA, INC.**
3636 Sixteenth St., N.W.
WASHINGTON, D.C.
20010

**CHARLES PARK**
446 Albert St.
LIMA, OHIO
45804

**PHILLIPS PETROLEUM CO.**
Editorial Division
4 A4 PB
BARTESVILLE, OKLA.
74004

**PLAYGROUND CORPORATION OF AMERICA**
29-24 40 Ave.
LONG ISLAND CITY, N.Y.
11101
   also
2298 Grissom Drive
ST. LOUIS, MO.
63141

(in Canada)
**PLAYSCAPES INTERNATIONAL**
Suite 1007—Dominion Square Bldg.
MONTREAL 110, P.Q., CANADA

**PLAYSKOOL—A MILTON BRADLEY CO.**
SPRINGFIELD, MASS.
01101

**POSTGRADUATE CENTER FOR MENTAL HEALTH**
Department of Community Services and Education
124 E. 28 St.
NEW YORK, N.Y.
10016

**THE PRESIDENT'S COMMITTEE
ON EMPLOYMENT OF THE HANDICAPPED**
WASHINGTON, D.C.
20210

**J. A. PRESTON CORP.**
71 Fifth Ave.
NEW YORK, N.Y.
10003

**THE PROPELLER CLUB OF THE UNITED STATES**
17 Battery Place
NEW YORK, N.Y.
10004

**REHAB AIDS**
Box 826
MIAMI, FLA.
33143

**REHABILITATION CENTER**
Hadley Regional Medical Center
KAYS, KANS.
67601

**REHABILITATION GAZETTE**
4502 Maryland Ave.
ST. LOUIS, MO.
63108

**MISS ANNE I. REMIS**
Special Class Teacher
City School District
ROCHESTER, N.Y.
14614

**RESEARCH CENTER**
School of Home Economics
University of Connecticut
STORRS, CONN.
06268

**ROBIN-AIDS, INC.**
3353 Broadway
VALLEJO, CALIF.
94590

**ROCKY MOUNTAIN DENTAL PRODUCTS CO.**
P.O. Box 1887
DENVER, COLO.
80201

**W. T. ROGERS CO.**
Box 4327
MADISON, WISC.
53711

**DR. ELMO ROUNDY**
270 SFIT
Brigham Young University
PROVO, UTAH
84601

**FRED SAMMONS, INC.**
Box 32
BROOKFIELD, ILL.
60513

**SANI-SEAT, INC.**
6005 N. Sauganash Ave.
Chicago, Ill.
60646

**SCHOLASTIC MAGAZINE AND BOOK SERVICES**
50 W. 44 St.
NEW YORK, N.Y.
10036

**SCHWINN BICYCLE CO.**
1856 N. Kostner Ave.
CHICAGO, ILL.
60639

**SCOTT FORESMAN AND CO.**
Advertising Department
1900 E. Lake Ave.
GLENVIEW, ILL.
60025
   also
1955 Montreal Road
TUCKER, GA.
30084
   also
11310 Gemini Lane
DALLAS, TEX.
75229
   also
99 Bauer Drive
OAKLAND, N.J.
07436
   also
855 California Ave.
PALO ALTO, CALIF.
94304

**SEARS ROEBUCK AND CO.**
d/708—Parent Medical Department
Attn: K. Billick, R.N.
3333 W. Arthington St.
CHICAGO, ILL.
60607

**SHELTON INDUSTRIES**
14942 Jackson St.
MIDWAY CITY, CALIF.
92655

**SHERFEY DENTMOBILE, INC.**
2266 Lloyd Center
PORTLAND, ORE.
97232

**SIECUS**
1855 Broadway
NEW YORK, N.Y.
10023

**SKILL DEVELOPMENT EQUIPMENT CO.**
1340 Jefferson N.
ANAHEIM, CALIF.
92806

**ANITA SLOMINSKI, O.T.R.**
Coordinator
Cerebral Palsy Clinic
Indiana University Medical Center
INDIANAPOLIS, IND.
46202

**SMALLEY & BATES, INC.**
88 Park Ave.
NUTLEY, N.J.
07110

**SOUTH CAROLINA DEPARTMENT
OF MENTAL RETARDATION**
2414 Bull St.
COLUMBIA, S.C.
29201

**SOUTHERN REGIONAL EDUCATION BOARD**
130 Sixth St., N.W.
ATLANTA, GA.
30313

**SOUTHWESTERN PUBLISHING CO.**
5101 Madison Road
CINCINNATI, OHIO
45227

**THE SPASTIC CENTRE OF NEW SOUTH WALES**
6 Queen St.
Mosman, 2088, N.S.W.
AUSTRALIA

**SPIELWAREN-HEMMELER AG**
Hintera Vorstadt 11
5000-Arau/Schweiz
SWITZERLAND

**SPIES TRADING CO.**
75 Valentine Road
BLOOMFIELD, N.J.
07003

**SPOKEN ARTS, INC.**
310 N. Ave.
NEW ROCHELLE, N.Y.
10801

**STAINLESS MEDICAL PRODUCTS**
3107 S. Kilson Drive
SANTA ANA, CALIF.
92707

**STALL & DEAN MANUFACTURING COMPANY, INC.**
P.O. Box 698
95 Church St.
BROCKTON, MASS.
02401

**STATE UNIVERSITY CONSTRUCTION FUND**
194 Washington Ave.
ALBANY, N.Y.
12210

**STEPHEN FOSTER MEMORIAL**
University of Pittsburgh
PITTSBURGH, PA.
15213

**CHRISTINE STEPHENS, OTR**
Montebello State Hospital
BALTIMORE, MD.
21218

**R. H. STONE PRODUCTS**
18279 Livernois
DETROIT, MICH.
48221

**SUN PRODUCTS CORP.**
P.O. Box 150
BARBERTON, OHIO
44203

**SUPERIOR COACH DIVISION**
Sheller-Globe Corp.
1200 E. Kibby St.
LIMA, OHIO
45802
   also
**SHELLER-GLOBE**
Superior Southern Division
1 Superior Drive
KOSCIUSKO, MISS.
39090

**TEACHERS COLLEGE PRESS**
1234 Amsterdam Ave.
NEW YORK, N.Y.
10027

**TEACHING RESOURCES CORP.**
100 Boylston St.
BOSTON, MASS.
02116

*TODAY'S CHILD* **NEWS MAGAZINE**
Morton Edwards, Editor
School Lane
ROOSEVELT, N.J.
08555

**THE TOWER COMPANY, INC.**
5421 First Ave. S.
SEATTLE, WASH.
98108

**TRANS-AID CORP.**
20314 S. Tajauta Ave.
CARSON, CALIF.
90746

**TRAVELODGE INTERNATIONAL CORP.**
Box 308
EL CAJON, CALIF.
92022

**UNESCO GIFT COUPON OFFICE**
Room 2201
United Nations
NEW YORK, N.Y.
10017

**UNITED CEREBRAL PALSY ASSOCIATIONS, INC.**
66 E. 34 St.
NEW YORK, N.Y.
10016

**UNITED CEREBRAL PALSY ASSOCIATION
OF NEW YORK STATE**
815 Second Ave.
NEW YORK, N.Y.
10017

**UNITED CEREBRAL PALSY ASSOCIATION
OF WESTERN NEW YORK, INC.**
100 Leroy Ave.
BUFFALO, N.Y.
14214

**UNITED CEREBRAL PALSY OF DENVER, INC.**
2727 Columbine
DENVER, COLO.
80205

**UNITED CEREBRAL PALSY
OF NORTHWESTERN PENNSYLVANIA**
2230 Broad St.
ERIE, PA.
16503

**USOE/MSU REGIONAL INSTRUCTIONAL
MATERIALS CENTER FOR HANDICAPPED
CHILDREN AND YOUTH**
College of Education
218 Erickson Hall
Michigan State University
EAST LANSING, MICH.
48823

**VISUAL PRODUCTS**
3M Company
2501 Hudson Road
ST. PAUL, MINN.
55119

**VOCATIONAL GUIDANCE AND
REHABILITATION SERVICES**
Rehabilitation Center
2239 E. 55 St.
CLEVELAND, OHIO
44103

**THE VOICESPONDENCE CLUB**
P.O. Box 207
SHILLINGTON, PA.
19607

**SCULLY WALTON**
505 E. 116 St.
NEW YORK, N.Y.
10029

**JAY L. WARREN, INC., AUDITORY
TRAINING EQUIPMENT**
721 West Belmont
CHICAGO, ILL.
60657

**WARREN PAPER-BUILT-RITE TOYS**
3200 S. St.
LAFAYETTE, IND.

**DR. H. J. WATERS**
Kansas State Teachers College
EMPORIA, KANS.
66801

**ROBERT L. WEBB, EDITOR**
PARAPLEGIA NEWS
935 Coastline Drive
SEAL BEACH, CALIF.
90740

**WHEELCHAIR ELEVATORS, INC.**
P.O. Box 489
BROUSSARD, LA.
70518

**BRUCE A. WILSON**
Public Relations
The Cleveland Electric Illuminating Co.
P.O. Box 5000
CLEVELAND, OHIO
44101

**E. P. WOOTEN, PH.D.**
Physical Education for Exceptional Students
Gerlinger Annex, University of Oregon
EUGENE, ORE.
97403

**THE WRITER, INC.**
8 Arlington St.
BOSTON, MASS.
02116

**WRITERS' DIGEST**
22 E. 12 St.
CINCINNATI, OHIO
45210

# Index

Page numbers in *italics* indicate illustrations. Page numbers followed by the letter "t" indicate tabular material.

*Cover design and text layout by Patrick H. Turner*
*Composed by American Book–Stratford Press, Inc.*
*Printed by Murray Printing Co.*
*Harper & Row, Publishers*

*74 75 76 10 9 8 7 6 5 4 3 2*